Ear, nose and throat disorders

Library of General Practice   Vol. 10

Editorial Board

Chairman
John Fry   OBE MD FRCS FRCGP

James D.E. Knox   MD FRCP FRCGP
M. Keith Thompson   FRCGP DObstRCOG
John H. Walker   MD FFCM FRCGP DPH
Ian M. Stanley   MD ChB MRCP FRCGP

Vol. 1   **Hypertension**   *J. Tudor Hart*
Vol. 2   **The First Year of Life**   *G. Curtis Jenkins & R. Newton*
Vol. 3   **Rheumatology in General Practice**   *M. Rogers & N. Williams*
Vol. 4   **Renal Medicine and Urology**   *D. Brooks & N. Mallick*
Vol. 5   **The Use of Computers in General Practice**   *J. Preece*
Vol. 6   **Sexual Medicine**   *G.R. Freedman*
Vol. 7   **The Care of the Elderly in General Practice**   *M. Keith Thompson*
Vol. 8   **Respiratory Disorders**   *J. Fry, R. White & H. Whitfield*
Vol. 9   **Towards Better Practice**   *P. Martin, A. J. Moulds & P.J.C. Kerrigan*

Forthcoming volumes in the series

Ischaemic Heart Disease   *P. Dootson & D. Rowlands*
Anxiety and Depression   *J. Grabinar & M. Lader*
The GP and the Laboratory   *R.A.M. Oliver, W.R.G. Thomas & T.R. Tickner*
Gastrointestinal Disorders   *D.A. Coffman, L.J. Chalstrey & G. Smith-Laing*
Gynaecology and Obstetrics in General Practice   *J.W. Eddy & J.D. Owen*

The **Library of General Practice** is a series of books for GPs about medical problems as they present in the community. The editorial board is chaired by John Fry, OBE, MD, FRCS, FRCGP — himself a GP and also an experienced author and researcher and a member of the Council of the Royal College of General Practitioners.

Each volume deals with an important aspect of general practice, written by a GP well-known for his work in the field, often in association with a leading specialist in the field.

Practice Library said of the first volume in the series:
'. . . **if they are all equally good, this series will be a very important contribution to the educational material available in the general practice field . . .**'

If you would like further information on any of the titles, or details on how to order them, please write to:

Library of General Practice, Sales Promotion Department, Churchill Livingstone, Robert Stevenson House, 1-3 Baxter's Place, Leith Walk, EDINBURGH, EH1 3AF, UK

Ear, Nose and Throat Disorders

Gordon W. Hickish
VRD MB ChB FRCGP DCH
General Practitioner, Bransgore, Hampshire; GP Tutor,
Southampton University Faculty of Medicine; Hospital Practitioner,
ENT Department, St Bartholemew's Hospital, London

CHURCHILL LIVINGSTONE
EDINBURGH LONDON MELBOURNE AND NEW YORK 1985

CHURCHILL LIVINGSTONE
Medical Division of Longman Group Limited

Distributed in the United States of America by
Churchill Livingstone Inc., 1560 Broadway, New
York, N.Y. 10036 and by associated companies,
branches and representatives throughout the
world.

©Longman Group Limited 1985

All rights reserved. No part of this publication
may be reproduced, stored in a retrieval system,
or transmitted in any form or by any means,
electronic, mechanical, photocopying, recording or
otherwise, without the prior permission of the
publishers (Churchill Livingstone, Robert
Stevenson House, 1-3 Baxter's Place, Leith Walk,
Edinburgh, EH1 3AF).

First published 1985

ISBN 0 443 02977 6
ISSN 0263-9742

British Library Cataloguing in Publication Data
Hickish, Gordon W.
 Ear, nose and throat disorders.—(Library
of general practice ISSN 0263-9742)
 1. Otolaryngology
 I. Title   II. Series
 617'.51   RF46

Library of Congress Cataloging in Publication Data
Hickish, Gordon W.
 Ear, nose and throat disorders
 (Library of general practice, ISSN 0263-9742;
vol. 10)
 Includes index.
 1. Otolaryngology. I. Title. II. Series: Library
of general practice; v. 10. [DNLM: 1. Otorhino-
laryngologic Diseases. W1 L102C v.10/WV 100
H628e] RF46.H53 1985 617'.51 84-21440

Produced by Longman Group (FE) Limited
Printed in Hong Kong

To Aileen

Note

Our knowledge in clinical medicine and related biological sciences is constantly changing. As new information obtained from clinical experience and research becomes available, changes in treatment and in the use of drugs become necessary. The author and the publisher of this volume have, as far as it is possible to do so, taken care to make certain that the doses of drugs and schedules of treatment are accurate and compatible with the standards generally accepted at the time of publication. The readers are advised, however, to consult carefully the instruction and information material included in the package insert of each drug or therapeutic agent that they plan to administer in order to make certain that there have been no changes in the recommended dose of the drug or in the indications or contraindications for its administration. This precaution is especially important when using new or infrequently used drugs.

Foreword

Prior to 1950 there existed in this country an abysmal lack of authoritative text books on diseases of the ear, nose and throat, apart from the famous 'Nose and Throat' of Sir St Clair Thomson and Negus, and that equally well known volume of Logan Turner from North of the Border.

The post-war decade saw a number of new books in the specialty, but these fell mainly into two categories. Some were immense tomes aimed at fully-fledged or embryo specialists and others were slick little handbooks to aid undergraduates in their exams.

At long last has arrived a book which must be the answer for that vast army of dedicated general practitioners who, whilst wishing to give of their best, may realize that owing to the allotment of time to subject in the undergraduate curriculum, they are less at home with head-lamp and otoscope, than with stethoscope and sphygomanometer.

Dr Gordon Hickish, a general practitioner of long standing, has worked as a clinical assistant for many years in the Ear, Nose and Throat Department of St Bartholomew's Hospital. He is therefore in a fine position to see the various facets of the picture and his book is literally packed with information vital to his fellow practitioners.

Indeed, so informative in his exposition of the most important medico-sociological problems in our specialty, for example, noise induced hearing loss and deafness in childhood and old age, that there are few candidates for the higher examinations in otolaryngology who would not benefit by making a careful study of his book.

Devizes, Wiltshire   Miles Foxen
1985

Preface

I owe a very deep debt of gratitude to Mr Robin McNab Jones, Senior Surgeon, Ear, Nose, and Throat Department, St Bartholomew's Hospital, for agreeing to act as Specialist Adviser in the preparation of this book. He read the manuscripts, and his many constructive criticisms and kindly guidance made my task not merely possible but a joy.

Treatment of many disorders encountered in general practice has yet to be placed on a sound scientific footing — largely for lack of knowledge of the natural history of diseases and of the effectiveness and risks of available therapeutic measures. Examples of such conditions in the ENT field include 'glue' ear, recurrent otitis media, and Menière's disease — and for similar reasons the indications for antibiotic administration, tonsillectomy, and other measures, remain controversial.

However, the scene is set for much of this uncertainty to be dispelled. All newly appointed principals in general practice are now vocationally trained; a growing number of practices are being upgraded to qualify as training practices — with implications so far as record keeping, age/sex registers, and staffing are concerned; more practices are installing computers; and many of the most able graduates are being attracted into general practice.

One task awaiting family doctors in this new era is the collection of epidemiological and clinical data needed, so that advice on management, based on a sounder scientific foundation, can be more confident in the future.

Bransgore, Hampshire   Gordon Hickish
1985

Acknowledgements

Apart from providing material acknowledged in the text, many people helped me in the preparation of this book.

I am indebted to Mrs Kriya Walmsley and Mrs Pat Butler who typed and re-typed the manuscript and the index respectively.

Dr Valerie Cleaver, Hearing Therapist, Royal Victoria Hospital, Bournemouth; Dr Pamela Ewan, Senior Lecturer in Clinical Immunology, St Mary's Hospital, London; and Dr Lynn Josephs gave me valuable advice.

The help I received from the staff of the Medical College Library and the Department of Audiology at St Bartholomew's Hospital has been greatly appreciated. A. H. Robins Company, Limited, generously made it possible to include the colour illustrations.

Last, but not least, I am beholden to Dr John Fry for his example and for effectively commissioning this volume, and to Mr Lance Dowie, Surgeon-in-Charge, ENT Department, St Bartholomew's Hospital, for introducing me to 'ENT'.

Contents

Part 1. General   1

1. Introduction   3
2. Essentials of ENT examination in general practice   5

Part 2. The ear   13

3. External ear disorders   15
4. Middle ear disorders   26
5. Deafness   63

Part 3. The nose   131

6. Anatomy and examination of the nose   133
7. Upper respiratory tract infections   138
8. Vasomotor rhinitis   152
9. Nasal polypi   163
10. Epistaxis   165
11. Injuries to the nose and snoring   170

Part 4. The pharynx and larynx   173

12. Anatomy and examination of the pharynx and larynx   175
13. Tonsil and adenoid problems   186
14. Croup and hoarseness   199
15. Dysphagia   208

Index   214

Part 1
General

1
Introduction

Diseases of the ear, nose, and throat form a substantial part of the general practioner's workload. Statistics published jointly by the Royal College of General Practitioners, Office of Population Censuses and Surveys, and Department of Health and Social Security indicated that even after common colds and acute sore throats are excluded, 7% of the episodes of disease seen in general practice are are due to ear nose and throat (ENT) problems.

Unfortunately, at present, preparation for care of ENT conditions seems neglected, relative to their importance, both at undergraduate and at postgraduate stages of medical education. A survey (Morris & Pracy 1983) of 24 medical schools in the United Kingdom, conducted by Sir Douglas Ranger, indicated an average undergraduate period of only 49 hours devoted to the speciality (at one the figure was 19 hours). Little of the subject is learnt during the pre-registration year, for the General Medical Council does not recognise pre-registration posts in otorhinolaryngology as providing adequate surgical experience. Of the 207 bodies organising vocational training for general practice in England and Wales, only 36 (17%) offer senior house officer posts in ENT in any of their schemes (Vocational Training Schemes for General Practice, 1982).

An audit of ENT referrals (Knowles et al, 1979) in the Boston area of Lincolnshire identified failure to ask relevant questions, and unsatisfactory examination technique, as the main deficiencies in general practice.

Judging from the multitude of questions raised at vocational training day release course sessions devoted to disorders of the ear, nose, and throat, trainees in general practice are well aware of these shortcomings in teaching and experience, and are eager to remedy them.

A characteristic of ENT work is that correct diagnosis rests largely on the doctor's capacity to see into dark cavities. Success depends both on competence and the availability of a minimum of basic equipment. Some of the unsatisfactory examination techniques noted in the Boston audit doubtless arose because general practitioners were working with equipment and illumination of a standard poor enough to have daunted a specialist.

REFERENCES

Knowles J E A, Savory J N, Royle R A, Deacon S P 1979 An audit of ENT referrals assessing training needs for general practice trainees. Journal of the Royal College of General Practitioners 29 (209): 730–732

Morris P D, Pracy R 1983. Training for ENT problems in general practice. The Practitioner 227: 995–999

Vocational training schemes for general practice 1982, 4 Edition. Published by the council for postgraduate medical education in England and Wales. 7 Marylebone Road London NW15HH

2
Essentials of ENT examination in general practice

Satisfactory examination of the ear, nose and throat depends both on brightness of illumination of the subject, and on exclusion of excessive background illumination. The latter requirement is basic – nobody would expect the cinema lights to be kept on during the showing of a film – yet often neglected. An area in the consulting room should be selected for ENT (and ophthalmological) examination, away from bright sunlight and capable of being further darkened, by extinguishing lights and drawing curtains or blinds, when necessary.

Every general practitioner uses an electric otoscope (auriscope) and the best results are obtained in subdued light. Illumination has traditionally been by means of an electric bulb set into the otoscope so that the examiner looks down the beam. In recent years fibroptically illuminated otoscopes have been introduced in which light is carried down a sheath of fibres, the ends of which form a ring round the speculum tip (Fig. 2.1). As a consequence the tympanic membrane is 'flood-lit'. In the healthy ear the tympanic membrane is thin and semi-transparent. It is possible, using a 'traditional' otoscope, to discern, through the tympanic membrane, the outline of the long process of the incus, running downwards parallel with, behind, and deep to the handle of the malleus (Fig. 2.2). This is a most useful pointer that the tympanic membrane is normal and that the middle ear cavity contains air and not fluid. A disadvantage of the 'fibroptic' otoscope is that reflected light from the evenly illuminated tympanic membrane makes this assessment difficult.

Specula of assorted sizes should be available, and the largest which will fit the meatus comfortably should be used.

One decision to be reached by each general practitioner is whether he wishes to be able to work with both hands free. If so,

6   EAR, NOSE AND THROAT DISORDERS

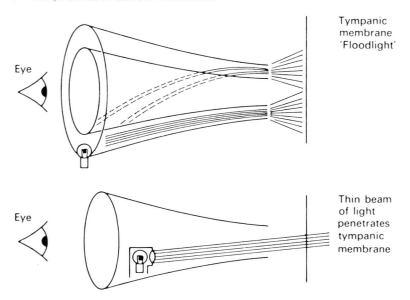

Fig. 2.1. Fibroptic (top) and 'traditional' (bottom) illumination systems.

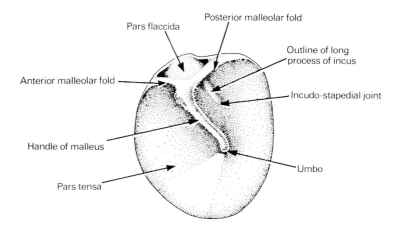

Fig. 2.2. (a) Normal ear (see plate section).
(b) Sketch of normal tympanic membrane (left).

a head mirror – or head worn lamp – will be required.

A head mirror has to be used in conjunction with a light source. The traditional 'Chiron' bull's eye lamp (Fig. 2.3) has been superceded by a halogen lamp, available from Downs Surgical In-

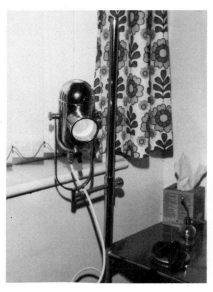

Fig. 2.3. Chiron lamp for use with head mirror.

struments, Church Path, Mitcham, Surrey CR4 3UE (current price £440–15p). A reflector-backed bulb in an 'anglepoise' type lamp is very much cheaper, and quite satisfactory.

When using a head mirror the light source should be just above the patient's left shoulder. The head mirror is worn so that the examiner looks through the central aperture with his right eye (if right handed), and should be as close to the eye as possible. The mirror diameter is small enough not to obstruct vision from the left eye, and this eye should be kept open as it contributes some useful orientation.

An alternative to a light source and head mirror is a head worn lamp (Fig. 2.4). This is inexpensive – it may be powered from a transformer often already available in the practice for electrocautery – and has many advocates (Horsfull, 1981). A disadvantage is that once 'wired up' the examiner's mobility is restricted.

Many general practitioners 'get by' when examining the ear, nose, and throat, equipped solely with a pen torch and otoscope. However, furnished with a head mirror or head worn lamp so that both hands are free (one to hold the speculum whilst the other works with an instrument) it is possible to do much more for the patient. In the ear, external meati and mastoid cavities can be

8 EAR, NOSE AND THROAT DISORDERS

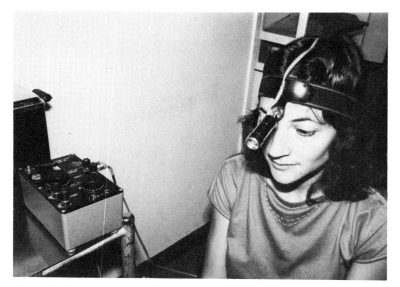

Fig. 2.4. Head-worn lamp with transformer.

cleaned, medications applied and wicks inserted under direct vision. In the nose, much fuller examination for such conditions as polyps or septal deviations is possible, and epistaxes from Little's area can be cauterised, and foreign bodies removed. In the throat, thorough examination under direct vision is possible, and using a mirror, the post nasal space (p. 136), hypopharynx, and larynx (p. 183) may be inspected.

INSTRUMENTS

The following instruments are desirable.

Ear

1. Jobson Horne probe, to hold cotton wool pledgets for cleaning the ear and applying medication (Figs 2.5 & 2.7).
2. Wax Hook: the St Bartholomew model is ideal (Figs 2.6 & 2.7).
3. Angled forceps (Fig. 2.7).
4. Small crocodile forceps for grasping objects within the meatus. Quire's forceps are satisfactory and much less expensive than other models (Fig. 2.7).

GENERAL PRACTICE EXAMINATION 9

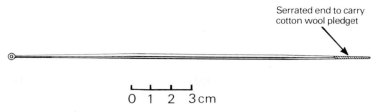

Fig. 2.5. Jobson Horne probe.

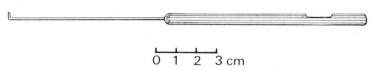

Fig. 2.6. Wax hook. Bartholomew model.

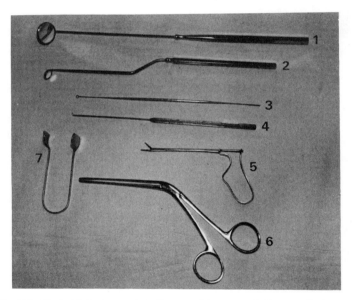

Fig. 2.7. Desirable instruments in the consulting room. 1. Laryngeal mirror; 2. post-nasal mirror; 3. Jobsen Horne probe; 4. Bartholomew wax hook; 5. Quire's torceps; 6. Angled forceps; 7. Thudichum's speculum.

5. Inflation bulb (Fig. 2.8). Most electric otoscopes have a nipple for attachment of a rubber bulb. Capacity to vary pressure in the external meatus is invaluable in assessing mobility of the tympanic membrane and in distinguishing retraction pockets from perforations. Unfortunately bulbs supplied for use with

10   EAR, NOSE AND THROAT DISORDERS

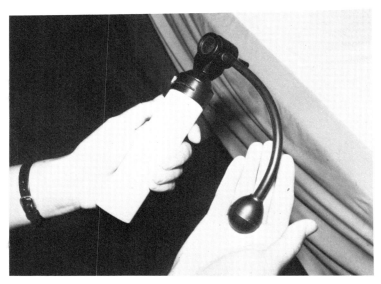

Fig. 2.8. Inflation bulb attached to electric otoscope.

electric otoscopes are usually so diminutive that only small pressure variations are possible and the examination is as a result often inconclusive. Greater pressure variations may be produced by sucking and blowing into a rubber tube attached to the otoscope (a method favoured in the USA).

6. Seigle's speculum (Fig. 2.9) is invaluable where a head mirror or head worn lamp is used. It consists of a chamber with a magnifying lens (set at an angle to avoid reflected light) at one end, and a rim for attachment of specula at the other.

A large inflation bulb attached to the chamber provides for effective inflation, and must be used gently to avoid causing pain.

7. Tuning fork (p. 72).
8. Ear syringe (p. 20).
9. Audiometer (p. 74).

Nose

Thudichum's specula (p. 136), preferably two or three sizes, are essential (Fig. 2.7).

An anaesthetic/vaso-constrictor spray such as 10% cocaine or Xylocaine spray is invaluable to shrink swollen nasal mucosa and permit instrumentation.

GENERAL PRACTICE EXAMINATION 11

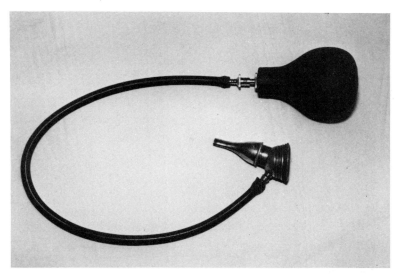

Fig. 2.9. Seigle's speculum

Caustics such as silver nitrate available ready impregnated on orange sticks (p. 167) or an electrocautery (p. 169) are required for treatment of epistaxis, together with a supply of ribbon gauze and BIPP paste (p. 166).

Throat

Tongue depressors. Wooden tongue depressors are widely used.

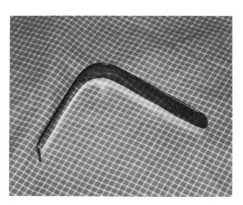

Fig. 2.10. Lack's tongue depressor.

Lack's angled metal tongue depressor has the advantage that the examiner's hand is out of the line of view (Fig. 2.10).

Post-nasal mirrors and laryngeal mirrors [two sizes: small (20 mm) for women and larger (30 mm) for men] should be sterilised by immersion in spirit or Hibitane and never boiled, as this will cause them to tarnish rapidly.

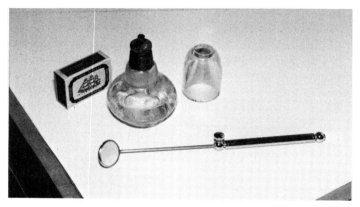

Fig. 2.11. Spirit lamp with laryngeal mirror.

A spirit lamp (Fig. 2.11) is valuable to heat the mirror before use to prevent condensation (and also serves other purposes in the consulting room). Care must be taken that it is charged with industrial or methylated spirit and never with surgical spirit which gives an inadequate flame and burns to produce offensive fumes.

REFERENCES

Horsfall T J M 1981 Instruments for examining the ear. Update 23 (7): 897–898

Part 2
The Ear

3
External ear disorders

ANATOMY

The skin of the pinna is closely attached to the underlying perichondrium except at the lobule and along the helix (Fig. 3.1).

The external meatus, about 25 mm long in adults, consists of an outer cartilaginous one-third and an inner bony two-thirds. The outer one-third is lined by skin 1–1.5 mm thick containing many sebaceous and ceruminous glands. Many hair follicles are present,

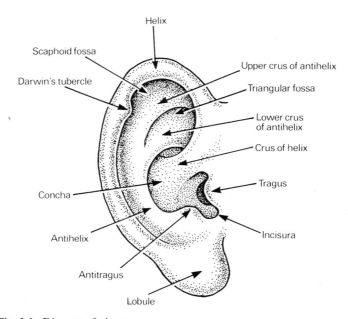

Fig. 3.1. Diagram of pinna.

and the hairs (vibrissae) become luxuriant in males after the age of 40 years.

The skin of the inner two-thirds of the external meatus is only 0.1 mm thick, closely attached to underlying periosteum, and extremely sensitive. Hairs, sebaceous and cerumenous glands are absent (Fig. 3.2).

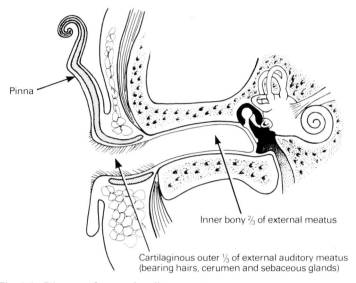

Fig. 3.2. Diagram of external auditory meatus.

Epithelial migration

The external auditory meatus is normally kept clean by epithelial migration. Growth begins at the umbo at the centre of the tympanic membrane, and surface cells pass centrifugally to the periphery of the drum, then outwards along the external meatus at a rate of about 0.05 mm day. Any foreign material in the meatus is carried outwards on this epithelial 'conveyor belt'.

DISORDERS OF THE PINNA

Otitis externa

This may involve the pinna and/or the external meatus, and may be one of the following:

a. Essentially a localised eczema.
b. Part of a more generalised skin disorder such as atopic eczema, seborrhoeic dermatitis or psoriasis.
c. A contact dermatitis. Hair lacquer, chemical constituents of hearing aid inserts, and topical antibiotics, particularly neomycin, are common culprits.
d. Infective, from bacterial, viral, or fungal agents. Secondary bacterial infection frequently complicates types a, b, and c.
e. As with other dermatoses, emotional factors may play an important part.

Otitis externa of the pinna leads to inflammation with thickening, local heat, redness, and often excoriation and weeping of serous fluid, with irritation and soreness. Postauricular eczma may occur alone or as part of a widespread flexural eczema, and may be missed unless the pinna, which may appear normal, is folded forwards.

Trauma

Sub-perichondrial haematomas result from injury to the pinna: boxers and rugby forwards are particularly at risk. Left untreated, cartilage degeneration and organisation of the haematoma are likely to occur, resulting in 'cauliflower ear' deformities. The haematoma should be aspirated through a wide bore needle and a pressure dressing applied, with padding behind the ear and in the concha, to discourage recurrence of the haematoma.

Chondrodermatitis (nodularis chronicis helis)

This is a painful condition of the helix, usually affecting the upper part, in which an area of cartilage and overlying skin becomes hot, red, swollen, tender and very painful. It is commonest in men of middle age or older, and vaso-constriction from cold exposure is often held responsible. The lesions may be sufficiently distressing to warrant excision.

Solar keratoses and basal cell carcinomas

These are liable to develop on the pinna as a result of its exposed situation. Solar keratoses may be destroyed with electro-cautery under local anaesthesia. Basal cell carcinomas are usually best referred to a plastic surgeon for treatment.

Congenital malformations

The pinna develops as a result of union of six rudimentory cartilaginous tubercles. Whilst gross deformities, such as anotia or microtia are rare, less severe malformations, particularly 'bat ear' are quite common.

Since the otic capsule, from which the inner ear develops, is formed earlier than and independently of the outer and middle ears, even gross pinna malformations may be associated with a normal labyrinth and useful hearing may be possible albeit sometimes with the help of reconstructive surgery.

Bat ear

This is the commonest ear malformation calling for plastic surgery (Fig. 3.3). An elipse of skin and cartilage is excised from behind the pinna, and closure of the wound draws the auricle inwards to a normal position close to the head. Boys with bat ear deformities are liable to be ridiculed at school, and surgical correction is best carried out before school age if possible. Unfortunately the cartilage of the pinna is sometimes insufficiently stiff for operation to be feasible until the age of 7 or 8 years. Girls are more able to conceal

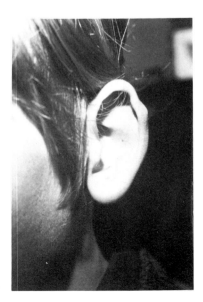

Fig. 3.3. Bat ear.

the malformation until later childhood, and may not present for operation until they wish to wear their hair up.

DISORDERS OF THE EXTERNAL AUDITORY MEATUS

Wax

Wax is formed from the combined secretions of the sebaceous and ceruminous glands of the outer third of the external auditory meatus. People of Caucasian and Negro race tend to make thin sticky wax, whilst mongoloid people more often have dried hard wax. The characteristics of forming 'wet' and 'dry' wax is inherited as an allelomorphic pair, the 'wet' gene being dominant over the 'dry'. The full implications of this distinction are still uncertain, but there is evidence suggesting that 'dry' wax makers enjoy some protection from respiratory infections.

A ring of wax round the outer one-third of the external auditory meatus serves as a protection against entry of foreign particles, bacteria, and insects into the deeper meatus. Wax normally dries and is continuously and imperceptibly shed as a powder, new formation and shedding keeping pace. Accumulation of wax is often the result of frequent wetting of the ears during washing. Some patients appear to make excessive quantities of wax, and wax accumulation is sometimes due to peculiarities of shape of the external auditory meatus.

Wax removal

Wax plugs of firm consistency are most simply and quickly removed with a wax hook. The St Bartholomew model is ideal. Using a head mirror or head-worn lamp, one hand is freed to manipulate the pinna to straighten the external meatus and to hold a speculum (the largest introducible) whilst the other wields the hook. It is sometimes necessary to free the wax plug from the walls of the meatus: the ring end of a Jobson Horne probe is convenient for this. The hook is then introduced, flush with the meatal wall, past the plug, and rotated so that the wax is extracted as the hook is withdrawn.

Soft wax may be wiped away with cotton wool pledgets mounted on a Jobson Horne probe. Gentleness is essential during these procedures. Stimulation of the auricular branch of the vagus nerve, which supplies part of the external meatus, may initiate the cough reflex.

Syringing

Where a history of tympanic membrane perforation can be excluded, wax may be removed by syringing. Two types of syringe are available: Wood's metal 'cylinder and plunger', and Bacon's syringe consisting of a Higginson's syringe with a metal cannula. This type of syringe is easier to use if several extra feet of tubing are let in.

Both types are liable to malfunction. The plunger in Wood's syringers may jam in the cylinder, or the seal may fail so that water and air leaks past the plunger. Regular dismantling and application of silicone or soap to the side of the plunger helps to avoid these difficulties.

Valves in the Bacon type syringe tend to seize up, and are then very difficult to free.

Shaw & Russell (1980) introduced a polypropylene syringe of improved design [Fig. 5.6(a) p 73], eliminating these difficulties. Competitively priced, it can be strongly recommended*.

Water temperature for syringing should be near to blood heat to avoid induction of convection currents in the lateral semicircular canal with resultant giddiness: 37°C is recommended, and beginners should be encouraged to check the temperature with a thermometer.

Procedure

The patient's clothing is protected with a waterproof bib and he is asked to hold a receiver (kidney dish or Noott's tank) against his neck below the ear (usually the opposite hand is most convenient). The pinna is then lifted upwards and outwards to straighten the external auditory meatus, (Fig. 3.4) and a jet of water is squirted along the roof of the meatus until the wax is washed out. The meatus should be inspected periodically with an auriscope during syringing. The tip of the syringe nozzle may be steadied against the outer meatus during syringing but should never be introduced into the deeper meatus. Varying the angle of the jet may help dislodge recalcitrant pieces of wax.

* Available from Russell Instruments, PO Box 1, Clarkston, Glasgow G 76.

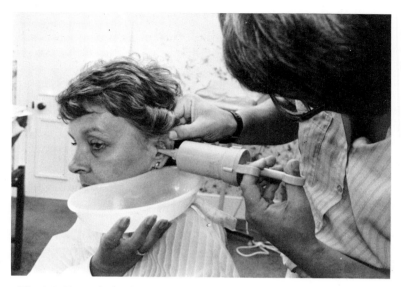

Fig. 3.4. Ear syringing in progress.

Once clean, the ear is tilted downwards to encourage the remaining water to run out, and the concha is dried with a tissue. The external meatus of patients subject to develop otitis externa should be mopped dry with cotton wool on a Jobson Horne probe.

Wax solvents

Wax too hard to be removed by syringing may be softened with solvent drops. Despite much experimentation no solvent has emerged of convincing superiority to Sodium Bicarbonate Ear Drops BPC (composed of sodium bicarbonate 5 g, glycerol 30 ml, and water to 100 ml). The British National Formulary recommends soaking cotton wool plugs in solvent and leaving them in the ear overnight for three nights before syringing.

Advantages of manual removal of wax

1. Safe in the presence of tympanic membrane weakness or perforation.
2. Usually quicker.
3. Appearance of tympanic membrane unaltered, facilitating subsequent examination.

4. Risk of precipitating otitis externa is avoided.

Syringing is a convenient means of removing wax in most cases, and has the advantage that the task may be delegated to a suitably trained assistant.

Otitis externa

Factors leading to otitis externa of the pinna (already considered) may also cause otitis externa of the external auditory meatus. In addition:

a. Failure of epithelial migration as a result, for example, of infection or wax accumulation, leads to accumulation of debris and to infection.
b. Misguided attempts to clean the external meatus are liable to cause trauma, predisposing to infection of the meatal skin.
c. Accumulated water behind a build-up of wax leads to maceration of the epidermis and to infection.
d. Discharge from a perforation of the tympanic membrane is commonly associated with otitis externa, whether or not the discharge is purulent.
e. The warmth and humidity of tropical climates favours development of otitis externa, particularly of fungal origin.

Diagnosis

Diagnosis is usually obvious from initial inspection but it may be difficult initially to ascertain whether or not there is an underlying otitis media.

Management

Ideally, a swab should be taken at the first encounter, and transferred to transport medium.

The meatus is then mopped clean using pledgets of cotton wool twisted onto a Jobson Horne probe. Clues as to aetiology may present during cleaning. Fungal infection from *Candida albicans* characteristically resembles wet blotting paper. In *Aspergillus niger* infection the black conidiophores are visible amongst the debris. *B. pyocyaneus*, *B. proteus*, and *Staph. aureus* are the commonest organisms encountered in diffuse otitis externa. A fishy odour points to

B. coli infection. A particularly evil smell suggests an underlying attico-antral chronic suppurative otitis media.

The presence of vesicles suggests viral infection.

Cleaning of the deeper part of the external auditory meatus requires patience and gentleness to avoid causing pain. Thorough cleaning of the external auditory meatus, usually repeated, may be the only treatment required for many cases of otitis externa.

Topical applications

These contribute to resolution and include the following.

1. Insufflated powders, such as chloramphenical powder, boric acid and iodine powder, Cicatrin powder or antifungal powders such as Clotrimazole 1% powder (Canesten).
2. Steroid ointments, of value in reducing inflammation and swelling. These are usually combined with 3.
3. Antibacterial and/or antifungal agents such as Triadcortyl (containing triamcinolone, nystatin, neomycin and gramicidin) or Dactacort (miconazole and hydrocortisone). A suitable mixture (for example of Locoid and Canesten ointment) may be made up at the time, a little of each being mixed, then applied on cotton wool mounted on a Jobson Horne probe like a paint.
4. Aqueous solutions containing steroid, antibiotics, and/or antifungal agents are widely used. Whilst they are undoubtedly often helpful, it seems in principle preferable to avoid water in the presence of otitis externa.

Prevention

Some patients appear particularly susceptible to otitis externa. As well as advising them to keep their ears dry, and to avoid traumatic attempts to clean the ears, the general practitioner can often help greatly by explaining the normal self cleansing of the external meatus through epithelial migration, and by advising the patient to report for cleaning of the meatus, initially at regular intervals of 2 or 3 months, and subsequently as soon as symptoms recur.

Furunculosis

Furunculosis begins as a staphylococcol infection of a hair follicle, and is consequently confined to the outer cartilagenous third of the external auditory meatus. Surrounding inflammation and oedema lead to blockage of the meatus, forward displacement of the pinna, and pain, considerably aggravated by manipulation of the pinna.

Treatment

This consists of systemic antibiotics, analgesia, and local measures.

A wick of ribbon gauze soaked in a steroid/antibiotic mixture (such as 'Terracortoril', Pfizer) gently introduced into the external auditory meatus reduces oedema and promotes drainage. The meatus should be mopped clean of purulent exudate once the furuncle has burst. In recurrent cases the urine should be checked for sugar and the anterior nares swabbed in case this is a reservoir of infection.

Foreign bodies

Small foreign bodies in the ear are usually conveniently removed by syringing. Larger foreign bodies, nearly filling the meatus lumen may merely be driven further and wedged by syringing. If of irregular shape, they may be grasped with crocodile or Quire's forceps, or extracted with a wax hook under illumination with a lamp and head mirror. No attempt should be made to grasp a large rounded foreign body with forceps owing to the risk of pushing it further in.

It is essential that the patient remain perfectly still during the removal of foreign bodies, and for many children and some adults this may entail hospital admission for general anaesthesia.

Exostoses (cold water swimmers' exostoses)

During routine examination of healthy adults rounded exostoses protruding into the external meatus lumen are sometimes seen (Fig. 3.5). Touching with a probe confirms their bony hardness. They appear to serve a protective function for the tympanic membrane and to develop in response to repeated immersion in cold water. Such exostoses seldom cause any inconvenience, and tend to regress if cold water swimming is discontinued.

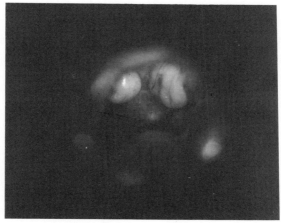

Fig. 3.5. Swimmer's exostoses.

Keratosis obturans

In this rare disease epithelial migration fails and the inner two-thirds of the external auditory meatus becomes blocked by an accumulation of desquamated squames resembling cholesteatoma. The obstructing material may enlarge, eroding into the surrounding bone. Initial cleaning may be difficult and require hospital admission for general anaesthesia. Thereafter the meatus must be inspected and cleaned every few months indefinitely.

Bullous (haemorrhagic) myringitis

In this viral infection of the tympanic membrane, sometimes encroaching onto the inner external meatal wall, large bullae often filled with bright red or dark blood are seen. The condition may be painful, but is self-limiting and the middle ear is usually unaffected. Follow up is desirable for 1 or 2 weeks until the tympanic membrane is seen to be returning to normal, but treatment is generally unnecessary.

4
Middle ear disorders

ANATOMY

The tympanic membrane (t.m.) dividing the external auditory meatus (e.a.m.) from the middle ear, consists of three layers: an outer epithelial and an inner mucosal layer, separated (except superiorly, in the pars flaccida — Shrapnell's membrane) by a fibrous layer. The latter, composed of circular and radial fibres, incorporates the handle of the malleus. The periphery of the t.m. is thickened into a fibrocartilaginous annulus which fits into a circular groove, the tympanic sulcus, in the tympanic ring of the temporal bone. Consequently the surgeon is able to dislodge the t.m. out of the tympanic sulcus, and later replace it, without tearing it.

The middle ear (Fig. 4.1) is a vertical cleft crossed by the chain of auditory ossicles: malleus, incus and stapes. Its shape resembles a biconcave disc 6 mm wide superiorly, 4 mm wide inferiorly, and only 2 mm wide in the centre. It communicates postero-superiorly, through the aditus, with the mastoid antrum and its associated air cells, and antero-inferiorly, via the Eustachian tube, with the postnasal space. Ciliated columnar epithelium lines the mucosa of the Eustachian tube and antero-inferior part of the middle ear, but gives way to thin cuboidal epithelium in the postero-superior part and mastoid. Scanty ciliated cells are present in the mastoid.

On the posterior wall of the middle ear cavity, just below the aditus, a bony prominence, the pyramid, gives attachment to the stapedius muscle whose tendon runs to the neck of the stapes. Anteriorly, above the opening of the Eustachian tube, the tendon of the tensor tympani muscle issues from a bony canal on its way to the malleus.

The middle ear cavity extends both higher and lower than the

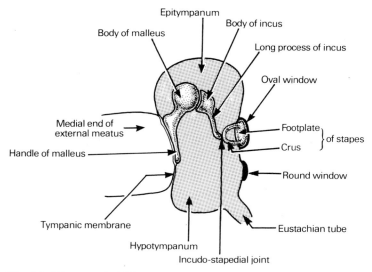

Fig. 4.1. Diagram of middle ear.

margins of the t.m. Above, the attic houses the head of the malleus and the body of the incus, and is separated from the middle cranial fossa by a thin plate of bone, the tegmen tympani. Below, the hypotympanum is separated by a thin plate of bone from the bulb of the jugular vein.

Much of the medial wall (Fig. 4.2) of the middle ear is visible in patients with large tympanic membrane perforations. The lowest turn of the cochlea produces a central elevation, the promontary. The oval window, containing the stapes footplate, lies above the promontary posteriorly. Below it is the round window closed by the secondary tympanic membrane. The facial nerve runs in the canal above the oval window, and higher up lies the anterior end of the lateral semicircular canal.

The chorda tympani, the chief nerve of taste, arises from the facial nerve just before it leaves the skull at the stylo-mastoid foramen. It runs forwards through the middle ear cavity, passing between the malleus and the incus, to enter a bony canal at the upper part of the anterior wall on its way to join the lingual nerve. As well as taste fibres, the chorda tympani conveys secretory fibres supplying the submandibular and sublingual salivary glands via the submandibular ganglion.

The tympanic plexus of nerves fibres lies beneath the mucosa of the medial wall of the middle ear. It is derived partly from the tym-

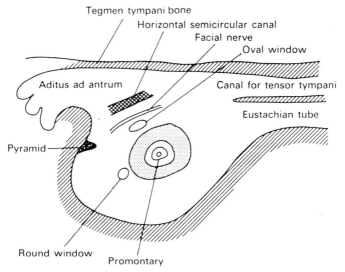

Fig. 4.2. Diagram of structures on medial wall of middle ear

panic nerve, a branch of the glossopharyngeal nerve, and partly from the sympathetic plexus around the internal carotid artery.

Fibres from the glossopharyngeal nerve include the following.
1. Sensory fibres to the mucous membrane of the Eustachian tube, middle ear and mastoid.
2. Secretory fibres to the parotid gland (travelling in the lesser superficial petrosal nerve to the otic ganglion where they synapse).

The chorda tympani and tympanic plexus are vulnerable to middle ear infection, trauma, or surgery, and the resultant disturbances of taste, salivation, and sensation may be very distressing.

Macewen's triangle (Fig. 4.3) is an important surface landmark: the mastoid antrum lies 1.5 cm deep to it in the adult, but is much more superficial in children. The triangle is bounded by the suprameatal crest above, the orifice of the external meatus anteriorly, and a vertical tangent to the posterior margin of the meatus posteriorly.

ACUTE OTITS MEDIA

Acute otitis media is very common: one in three children under 10 years of age in Britain have at least one attack (Fry 1972), and it causes much childhood misery.

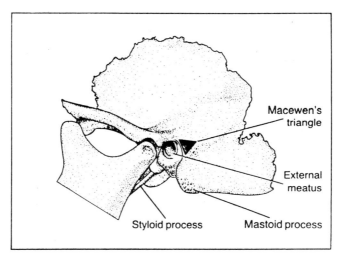

Fig. 4.3. Macewen's triangle is an important landmark. The mastoid antrum lies 1.5 cm deep to it in the adult, but is much more superficial in children. The triangle is bounded by the suprameatal crest above, the orifice of the external meatus anteriorly, and a vertical tangent to the posterior margin of the meatus posteriorly.

Epidemiology and pathogenesis

Acute otitis media almost always accompanies, or follows, an upper respiratory infection, and is most common in children aged 5–6 years (Fig. 4.4). Fry's studies (ibid, 1972) indicated 50–60 cases annually in a practice of 2500 patients. Statistics gathered by the Royal College of General Practitioners Birmingham Research Unit and the University of Surrey Epidemiological Observation Unit confirm a close relationship between the common cold and acute otitis media. Both are about three times commoner in winter than summer, and general practitioners see about two common colds for every case of otitis media.

Direct spread from the nasopharynx along the Eustachian tube is much the commonest route of entry, but entry of infection to the middle ear through a t.m. perforation can occur, as can involvement of the middle ear mucosa as part of a widespread viraemia.

In infants the Eustachian tube is relatively wide and straight, and milk or vomit may enter the middle ear setting up an initial 'chemical' otitis media which subsequently becomes secondarily infected.

30 EAR, NOSE AND THROAT DISORDERS

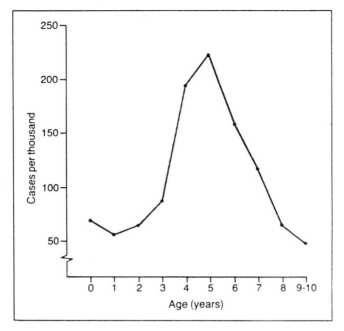

Fig. 4.4. Annual prevalence rates of acute otitis media (courtesy of Dr J. Fry).

Virology and bacteriology

It remains uncertain in what proportion of cases otitis media is

a. Purely viral,
b. Bacterial secondary to viral infection,
c. Due to bacterial invasion in the first place.

It seems reasonable to assume, since viral upper respiratory infection preceeds most cases of acute otitis media, that b is predominant. However attempts to isolate viruses from middle ear aspirates in acute otitis media are often unsuccessful. In one study of 663 aspirates (Klein & Teale, 1976) a virus was isolated in only 4.4%. Respiratory syncitial virus and influenza virus were the most common isolates, and were most often present during epidemics.

The low rate of isolation of viruses from middle ear aspirate in acute otitis media may indicate one of the following.

1. No virus was present.
2. Viruses were present earlier but are now absent.

3. Viruses are present in concentrations too low to identify by present techniques.
4. Inhibitors such as antibody, interferon, or lysozyme may prevent successful isolation of viruses.

Studies of middle ear aspirates from cases of acute otitis media consistently indicate *Haemophilus influenzae* and *Streptococcus pneumoniae* to be the commonest bacterial pathogens. *Staphylococcus pyogenes* is reported less commonly. 30 to 40 per cent of middle ear aspirates have yielded no bacterial pathogen.

Schwartz et al (1977) aspirated middle ear contents in 58 children aged 5–9 years with acute otitis media and found

H. influenzae in 36%,
Strep. pneumoniae in 24%,
Staph. pyogenes in 10%,
No bacterial pathogen in 30%.

Other workers have considered *Streptococcus pneumoniae* to be the commonest causative organism and recommend vaccination of infants and children with a pneumococcol vaccine after a first attack of acute otitis media (Makela & Karma, 1981).

Natural history

Infection is usually confined to the mucosa and submucosa of the middle ear which swell, blocking the Eustachian tube. Ciliary action is paralysed, and goblet cells increase. The t.m. loses its normal translucency and becomes reddened and opaque. Absorption of gas, particularly oxygen, in the non-ventilated middle ear cavity results in negative pressure which in turn promotes fluid transudation and draws the t.m. inwards. Increasing fluid transudation and inflammatory exudation finally cause bulging of the t.m.

Pain increases, and younger patients may be febrile and toxic.

Sometimes pressure necrosis and capilliary thrombosis lead to rupture of the drum, followed by purulent and often haemorrhagic otorrhoea, and by almost immediate pain relief. Usually resolution without t.m. rupture takes place over the course of 1 or 2 weeks and by 3–4 weeks appearances are back to normal. However effusion has been found to persist for 2 weeks in 50% of children, and still to be present after 6 weeks in 15% of these (Schwartz et al, 1981).

Clinical picture

The onset of earache in a patient with an upper respiratory tract infection is virtually diagnostic of otitis media, and otoscopy is usually merely a confirmatory measure.

Children are usually febrile. Toddlers too young to describe their symptoms are likely to be fretful or crying, and often put a hand to their ear. Babies may be merely 'off their feeds' and unsettled and may have vomiting and/or diarrhoea. Inspection of the t.m. is of course essential in any vaguely unwell infant.

Acute otitis media results in deafness, but this complaint is usually overshadowed by the pain.

Diagnosis

Initially injection of vessels along the handle of the malleus may be the only visible abnormality (Fig. 4.5). Soon the t.m. loses its greyish transparency and becomes opaque, red, and either indrawn or, more commonly, bulging with loss of landmarks (Fig. 4.6).

Inspection of the t.m. may be obstructed by wax and debris in the external meatus. Syringing to remove this is the presence of suspected otitis media is contra-indicated on account of pain and the risk of rupturing the t.m. Even gentle mopping may be quite agonising, and a provisional diagnosis based on the history and clinical picture is best acted upon and treatment begun. The diagnosis may be confirmed a few days later when acute inflammation has subsided and the meatus can be cleaned.

Instillation of a few sodium bicarbonate ear drops BPC often suffices to clean the e.a.m. adequately. At this stage the t.m. is likely to be opaque, dark in colour, and corrugated as a result of subsiding distension.

Management

Although no pathogenic bacteria can be cultured from middle ear aspirates in otitis media in some 30% of cases there is no way in which these, with a presumed viral aetiology, can be differentiated clinically from those associated with bacterial pathogens. Failure to treat bacterial infection adequately results in continuing pain, increased risk of t.m. perforation, damage to ossicles and their ligaments (likely to be followed by fibrosis and deafness), increased risk of serious complications such as mastoiditis, and increased likeli-

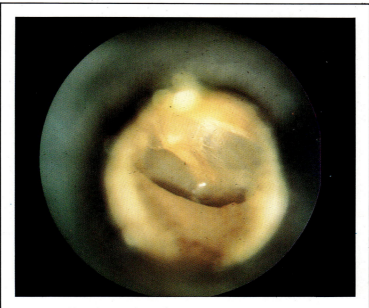

Fig 2.2(a) Normal tympanic membrane

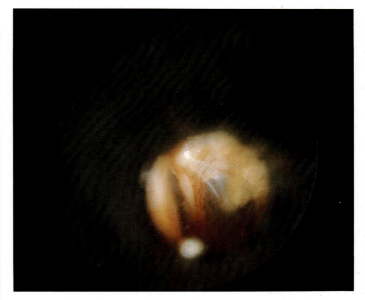

Fig 4.5 Early acute otitis media

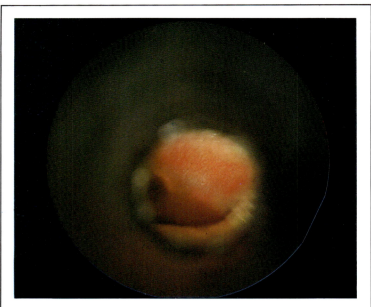

Fig 4.6 Acute otitis media

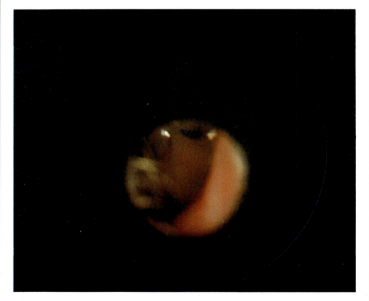

Fig 4.7 Glue ear

Table 1. Toxic reactions to antimicrobial agents.

Agent	Mechanism	Signs
Haematological		
Chloramphenicol	Inhibit protein synthesis	Reversible anaemia, leukopaenia
	Damage stem cell	Aplastic anaemia
Sulfonamides	G6PD deficiency	Hemolytic anaemia
Carbenicillin	Platelet aggregation inhibited	Bleeding
Nervous System		
Aminoglycosides	Binding hair cells or organ of Corti	Deafness
	Binding vestibular cells	Vertigo
	Competitive neuromuscular blockade	Respiratory paralysis
Polymyxins	Noncompetitive neuromuscular blockade	Respiratory paralysis
Penicillins and cephalosporins	Cortical stimulation	Myoclonic seizures
Gastrointestinal		
Rifampin	Liver cell damage	Hepatitis
Isoniazid		
Tetracycline		
Neomycin	Villi damage	Malabsorption
Clindamycin	Altered bowel flora – overgrowth *C. difficile*	Diarrhoea, pseudomembranous colitis
Lincomycin		
All agents	Altered bowel flora – overgrowth *C. difficile*	Diarrhoea, pseudomembranous colitis
Renal		
Penicillins	Interstitial nephritis	Fever, eosinophilia, azotaemia
Cephaloridine	Tubular necrosis	Azotaemia
Aminoglycosides	Tubular necrosis	Cylinduria, azotaemia
Metabolic		
Penicillins		
Carbenicillin	Nonabsorbable anion	Hypokalaemia
Ticarcillin		
Allergic		
Penicillins	IgE	Anaphylaxis
	IgM	Rash
Cephalosporins	?	Rash
Tetracyclines	?	Rash
Miscellaneous		
Cephalosporins		False-positive glucose tests

Table 2. Mechanism of action of antimicrobial agents.

Agents	Type of action	Site of action
1. β-Lactam antibiotics		
penicillins	Bactericidal	Cell wall
cephalosporins		
2. Vancomycin	Bactericidal	Cell wall
3. Aminoglycosides		
gentamicin		
tobramycin	Bactericidal	Protein synthesis
amikacin		
4. Erythromycin	Bacteriostatic	Protein synthesis
5. Clindamycin	Bacteriostatic	Protein synthesis
6. Tetracyclines	Bacteriostatic	Protein synthesis
7. Chloramphenicol	Bacteriostatic	Protein synthesis
8. Trimethoprim-	Together	Folic acid synthesis
sulfamethoxazole	bactericidal	
9. Rifampin	Bactercidal	RNA synthesis

Table 3. Micro-organisms involved in otolaryngological infections and agents which inhibit them.

Organism	Agents of choice
S. pneumoniae	Penicillins, cephalosporins, erythromycin
S. pyogenes	Penicillins, cephalosporins, erythromycin
S. aureus	Nafcillin, oxacillin, cloxacillin, cephalosporins
N. meningitidis	Penicillin
H. influenzae	Ampicillin, amoxicillin, cefaclor, cefamandole, trimethoprim sulfamethoxazole sulfamethoxazole
E. coli	Cephalosporins
Klebsiella	Cephalosporins, aminoglycosides
Pseudomonas	Carbenicillin, ticarcillin, tobramycin
B. fragilis	Clindamycin, chloramphenicol, cefoxitin
Anaerobic streptococci	Penicillins
Fusobacteria	Penicillins
B. melaninogenicus	Penicillins, erythromycin, clindamycin, cephalosporins

Reproduced by courtesy of Dr Harold Neu.

hood of recurrence. It therefore seems prudent to treat all cases of acute otitis media with antibiotics.

Antibiotic choice

Children

Since *Strep. pneumoniae* and most strains of *H. influenzae* are sensitive to Amoxycillin, this drug is suitable for initial therapy in acute otitis media.

Alternatively, Phenoxymethyl Penicillin (Penicillin 'V') remains highly effective for *Strep. pneumoniae* infections, which according to most studies is the commonest pathogen in acute otitis media. It is relatively ineffective against *H. influenzae*.

Where a good clinical response is not apparent by the second to third day on amoxycillin, a *H. influenzae* infection resistant to amoxycillin is likely to be present. A change to co-trimoxazole or cefaclor (Distaclor) is appropriate (other cephalosporins have poor activity against most strains of *H. influenzae*).

Adults

Oxytetracycline 250 mg four times/day is widely used, but penicillin, amoxycillin, co-trimoxazole or cefaclor may be preferred on account of the poor performance of tetracyclines against *Strep. pneumoniae*.

Duration of antibiotic therapy

Antibiotic administration for approximately 7 days is common practice and usually adequate.

However since effusion in the middle ear has been shown to persist after acute otitis media for several weeks (Shurin et al, 1979) and re-infection of persistent effusion may account for recurrence of acute otitis media during this time, continuation of antibiotic treatment for several weeks as a prophylactic measure has been advocated (Biedel. 1978) and should certainly be considered in children with repeated recurrences.

Analgesics

Analgesics are commonly needed during the early stages of acute otitis media. Aspirin is usually adequate.

Decongestant alpha-stimulator mixtures

Substances such as Dimotapp are commonly prescribed to promote Eustachian drainage, although scientific evidence supporting their effectiveness is lacking.

Myringotomy

This is nowadays seldom called for.

Perforation of the tympanic membrane

This affords an opportunity to swab and culture the middle ear contents so that subsequent antibiotic therapy may be soundly planned. Antibiotic drops, usually in conjunction with steroids, may be introduced into the middle ear through the perforation.

Follow-up

Ideally patients with acute otitis media should be re-examined on the second or third day to ensure that improvement is under way, with relief of pain and reduced inflammation. Where a change in antibiotic is made, a review after a further 2 to 3 days is called for.

At re-examination after 1 to 2 weeks the t.m. should no longer be inflamed. Hearing should be checked with whisper and tuning fork tests. Ideally, audiometry after 3 to 6 months should be performed (Fry, 1972).

Acute otitis media in presence of existing tympanic membrane perforation

Infection is likely to be due to organisms other than *Strep. pneumoniae* or *H. influenzae*, gaining entrance via the perforation. A bacterial swab should always be taken for culture and sensitivities.

Complications

Rupture of the t.m.

This is infrequent in cases treated with appropriate antibiotics. Most perforations heal leaving an insignificant scar, or no trace at all. Where infection has continued, and the perforation has persisted, final healing may result in a thin scar, the middle 'fibrous' layer of the t.m. failing to regenerate. Such thin scars may subsequently become 'indrawn' owing to negative middle ear pressure, laying the foundation for cholesteatoma formation. Thin scars are liable to break down easily, for example during ear syringing.

Recurrent otitis media

In a survey reported by Bain (1981) 25 general practitioners followed up 274 consecutive children with otitis media for 1 year; 43%

of the children had a recurrence, two-thirds of these occurring during the first 3 months.

In another study (Branefors-Hedlander et al, 1975) immunological and bacterialogical observations in a group of children with recurrent otitis media revealed the following.

1. No evidence of immunological deficiency to account for the recurrences.
2. In nearly every patient the organism responsible for a recurrence differed from that isolated at the previous infection; it was either a different organism or a different serological type of the same organism.

First encounter appears to be the predominant factor in recurrent otitis media. Where otitis media repeatedly recurs, management includes the following.

1. Attention to general health, nutrition, and possibly to environmental conditions.
2. Treatment of associated upper respiratory tract disorders including sinus, adenoid and tonsil infection sometimes calling for the help of an ENT surgeon.
3. Provision of antibiotic cover during acute upper respiratory infections.
4. Consideration of long-term antibiotic prophylaxis (by analogy with prophylaxis of bacterial endocarditis and pyelonephritis). Being inexpensive, relatively free from serious side effects, and effective against most strains of *H. influenzae* as well *Strep. pneumoniae*, Penicillin G orally has been advocated (Paradise, 1981)
5. Since *Strep. pneumoniae* is the commonest infecting organism in recurrent otitis media 14 – valent pneumococcal vaccine has been used to promote antibody production (Makela & Karma, 1981)
6. The effectiveness of long-term administration of decongestant – antihistamine mixtures (such as Dimotapp) has not been established by long-term double blind trials. Many doctors are sufficiently convinced of their value as to consider such trials unethical.

Chronic suppurative otitis media

This is a rare complication of adequately treated acute otitis media.

Acute mastoiditis

This has become a rarity in the antibiotic era. It is to be suspected when pain returns to an ear which has been discharging. Profuse offensive creamy discharge develops, deafness may increase, and the patient typically becomes pyrexial and toxic.

Infection has spread into the mastoid antrum and air cells, where thrombosis of small vessels results in necrosis. Oedema is often present over the mastoid, obliterating the post-auricular sulcus and pushing the pinna forwards. Movement of the pinna is not painful, in contradistinction to the extreme tenderness encountered in furunculosis of the external meatus which can lead to similar displacement of the pinna. Pain is felt on pressure over Macewen's triangle (Fig. 4.3). Mastoid X-ray reveals clouding of the mastoid system with decalcification and loss of cellular architecture.

Treatment of acute mastoidits

Hospital admission is necessary. Many cases respond to intensive intravenous chemotherapy. Subperiosteal collections of pus may be released by Wilde's incision. If clinical improvement is not evident within 24–48 hours, simple cortical or 'Schwartze' mastoidectomy is indicated (Fig. 4.14(a) p. 57). The mastoid antrum is entered through an incision over Macewen's triangle using an electric drill. All diseased mastoid cells are scraped away and small openings are made in the tegmen tympani above and the lateral sinus plate posteriorly to exclude extension of infection potentially leading to extradural abscess or lateral sinus thrombosis. Finally, the edges of the resulting bony pit are reduced for cosmetic reasons.

Masked mastoiditis

This condition, which is again rare, is to be suspected where acute otitis media fails to resolve normally, pain, pyrexia, and redness of the t.m. persist, and swelling and tenderness develop over the mastoid. X-rays again show clouding of the mastoid. Surgical drainage of both middle ear and mastoid are usually required.

Petrositis

Rarely, infection of air cells in the petrous temporal bone may lead to abscess formation near the apex. Pus may track outwards from the bone causing extradural abscess and meningitis. Infection at the petrous apex characteristically involves the overlying fifth nerve, causing deep temporal and retro-orbital pain, and the sixth nerve, paralysing the external rectus muscle; and there is usually an associated mastoiditis. The deep pain, sixth nerve palsy, and mastoiditis constitute Gradenigo's syndrome. Treatment involves antibiotics, mastoidectomy, and surgical drainage of the petrous abscess.

Zygomatic mastoiditis

This may occur where the zygoma is pneumatised and the overlying swelling may lead to confusion with mumps.

GLUE EAR

Secretory, serous, or 'non-suppurative' otitis media affects all age groups. In children the middle ear secretion shows a strong tendency to become thick, tenacious and glue-like. Jordan, of the USA, introduced the term 'glue ear' in the 1940s for this condition (Fig. 4.7).

Incidence

Serous otitis media is extremely common up to the age of 7 or 8 years. Studies indicate that newborn infants are unaffected, but that by the age of 1 year 14% of all ears have secretory otitis (Tos, 1981). In a group of toddlers examined five times during their third year only 23% were free of secretory otitis on all five occasions. 73% of 4-year-olds had secretory otitis media at at least one of five examinations (Tos et al, 1982). The observations were based on tympanograms (p. 43) and otoscopic examination. Indeed episodes of secretory otitis media would appear a 'normal' phenomenon in pre-school children and for the first 2 or 3 years of school life.

Natural history

In Lancashire, Hallett (1982) carried out tympanometry on a group of 553 5-year-old children in March, April, May, and November in 1980. At least 35% of the children had tympanometric evidence of middle ear disease in both ears on each occasion tested, yet by November, only 3% still had tympanometric evidence of middle ear disease in one or both ears.

Furthermore, the 35% with abnormal tympanograms during the monthly testings were not all the same children each time: there was a strong tendency for spontaneous improvement. Glue ear is a self limiting condition in the great majority of cases.

One or two per cent of adults have chronic otitis media. It seems likely that many if not most of these patients began with glue ear and have never acquired adequate Eustachian tube ventilation. Whether treatment can alter this progression remains uncertain. Mawson & Brennand (1969) considered that 10% of cases of glue ear referred to hospital will eventually need a hearing aid.

Aetiology

This remains uncertain but is probably multifactorial.

Allergy

Jordan (1969) considered that allergy played a large part. A retrospective study (Schutte et al, 1981) revealed a history of atopy to be twice as common in children with glue ear as in matched controls. Measurement of IgE specific to house dust mite and grass pollen revealed higher levels in children with glue ear than in a control group (Khan et al, 1981). The composition of middle ear effusion has been held to support a type III immune complex mechanism (Veltri & Sprinkle, 1976)

Infection

Fluid aspirated from the middle ear of patients with glue ear is most often sterile on bacterial culture, and efforts to isolate viruses have generally failed.

Although many believe that infection commonly plays a part in the initiation, if not the persistence, of glue ear, a history of documented acute otitis media is lacking in most glue ear sufferers. In a study of cultures of fluids aspirated from the ears of infants under the age of 1 year, the percentage of positive cultures fell as the age of the infant increased. At the same time the concentration of IgA and IgG increased. The findings support infection as an aetiological agent; the increase in immunoglobulins and decrease of positive cultures suggest that middle ear defence mechanisms develop with age (Juhn, 1982). A controlled trial of a 6 weeks course of Cotrimoxazole in serous otitis media in children under the age of 1 year showed a very clear benefit: 64% responded as against 26.9% in the control group (Marks et al, 1981)

Eustachian obstruction

Under normal conditions oxygen and nitrogen in the middle ear cavity diffuse into the mucosa creating slight negative pressure. The Eustachian tube is closed at rest. During swallowing contraction of the levator palati muscle, attached to the floor of the tube, causes the tube to open, and air passes to fill the relative vacuum in the middle ear. Children with cleft palates lack such normal levator palati function, and almost invariably suffer from glue ear.

Eustachian obstruction has been known for over two centuries to cause middle ear effusion (Wather, 1755). In animal experiments obstruction of the Eustachian tube leads to accumulation of serous fluid within 1 or 2 days.

In patients suffering from Eustachian obstruction, progressive negative pressure from air absorption results in serous transudate from mucosal capillaries. Anoxia of the epithelium impairs ciliary action and metaplasia occurs with increase in secretory and goblet cells. The character of the effusion subsequently changes, with increase in protein and potassium content, accumulation of cells including epithelial cells, lymphocytes and macrophages, and of enzymes (including dehydrogenases, alkali phosphatase and lysozyme), complement, prostaglandins, IgA, IgE, IgG, and IgM. Swelling of the Eustachian tube mucosa as a result of allergy or infection can produce obstruction. Hyperplasia of lymphoid tissue close to the Eustachian orifice (part of Waldeyer's ring) can also contribute. Enlarged adenoids are probably not an important cause of Eustachian obstruction. One recent study compared the size of adenoids of children with glue ear against those of matched controls and found no significant difference (Hibbert & Stell, 1982). Another (Maw et al, 1983) found no significant relationship between adenoidal volume and the presence or absence of middle ear fluid.

Resolution of glue ear results when aeration of the middle ear is restored, and is associated with return of the metaplastic mucosa to its normal histological state.

Consequences of glue ear

Although glue ear shows a strong tendency to spontaneous resolution after a variable period, affected children suffer a hearing loss whilst the condition persists. This may lead to slowing of educational advancement, noisy behaviour, impaired communication with family and friends, and has even been held responsible for childhood delinquency. Glue ear has also been considered the principal cause of dyslexia (Wisbey, 1982). Well managed glue ear appears to have no long-term effects (Hoffman-Lawless et al, 1981).

Recognition

The general practitioner is in an ideal position to recognise glue ear: a substantial proportion of children brought to him with upper respiratory infections and catarrh are likely to be suffering from it. Interest should be taken in siblings fortuitously attending the surgery. The noisy child who proceeds to dismantle one's equipment, heedless of his mother's entreaties, may well be affected. Recognition depends on a high index of suspicion, demonstration that hearing is impaired, and visualisation of the t.ms. Once a friendly rapport has been established, an effort to test the child's hearing should be made by whispering words familiar to him ('apples, oranges, bananas, sausages' or, in older children, numbers) at 1 m from each ear in turn, with the other ear covered. The child is asked to repeat the words if he hears them. In a quiet room he should be able to hear the faintest whisper.

Visualisation of the t.m.s. may require a little preliminary mopping of soft wax with cotton wool on a Jobson Horne probe. A practitioner familiar with the greyish transparent appearance of a normal t.m. will have little difficulty in recognising the dull, thickened, opaque, discoloured and often indrawn t.m. characteristic of glue ear. Observation during inflation (using the inflation bulb attached to the electric auroscope, or Seigle's speculum) helps to distinguish the normal 'mobile' t.m. from the t.m. immobilised by fluid beyond. A negative Rinne tuning fork test (p. 72) indicating conductive deafness in the presence of glue, completes the clinical examination of the ear.

The upper respiratory tract should also be examined generally for evidence of infection, allergy, or obstruction.

Audiometry

If an audiometer is available, and the child is old enough to co-operate whilst an audiogram is recorded, this is valuable. The severity of the hearing loss is documented, and a base line obtained for future comparison.

Tympanometry

Measurement of 'acoustic impedence' is used in audiology clinics to document negative middle ear pressure and the presence of middle ear fluid, and in some school clinics as a screening device for glue ear. The advantage of the method is that it is entirely objective.

An insert is placed in the external meatus, surrounded by a rubber collar so that an airtight seal is obtained. Three tubes run to the insert: one bringing sound signals, another leading to a microphone, and a third to a manometer and pressure regulator. The t.m. may be thought of as responding to sound signals by vibrating to a degree dependent on its compliance (the converse of impedence), which is maximal when the pressure either side of the t.m. is equal. The sound reflected from the t.m. is picked up by the microphone and measured. In the normal ear the air in the middle ear is at atmospheric pressure and when the pressure in the external meatus is adjusted to atmospheric, a maximum response is obtained. As the pressure is varied from atmospheric, the response becomes progressively weaker.

Acoustic impedence measurement is performed automatically by a 'middle ear analyser'. This instrument presents a repeated tone to the ear and records the reflected sound energy, as external meatal pressure is varied from negative to positive, in the form of a 'tympanogram' (Fig. 4.8).

Examples of a normal tympanogram, a tracing obtained in Eustachian dysfunction with negative middle ear pressure, and the flat tympanogram characteristic of glue ear are illustrated (Fig. 4.9).

It is customary at the conclusion of the tracing to deliver a loud sound to the ear and record the altered compliance produced by reflex contraction of the stapedius muscle. In the presence of glue, stapedius contraction has no measurable effect on compliance, and the tympanogram reveals absence of the stapedius reflex.

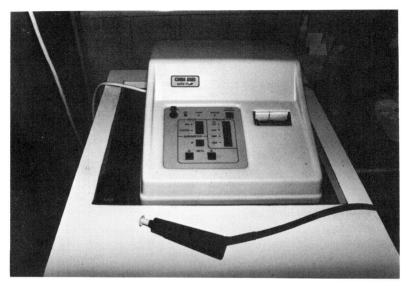

(a)

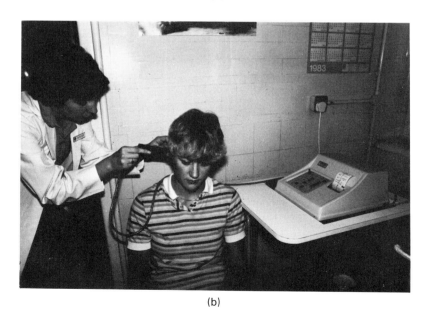

(b)

Fig. 4.8. Middle ear analyser. (a) Analyser with ear insert in Foreground. (b) Recording a tympanogram.

Screening for glue ear

The desirability of screening campaigns for glue ear in children of school age has been the subject of much debate. Mass screening, using the middle ear analyser, has been advocated. Some authorities consider the middle ear analyser too sensitive an instrument for screening, leading to the referral for further investigation of too large a proportion of children in whom no abnormality can subsequently be found (Hallett, 1982). Screening for stapedius reflex alone has been preferred (Brooks, 1976). However in the USA a panel of international authorities discussing screening for glue ear noted the continuing uncertainty surrounding the aetiology and advantages of treatment of the condition, and decided that it could not recommend mass screening by any method (Research conference on Recent Advances in Otitis Media with Effusion, 1980)

Management

Since the aetiology of glue ear remains uncertain, the condition usually resolves spontaneously, and possible long-term harmful effects of treatment have been a cause for concern, firm guidelines for management are difficult to construct. Treatments advocated include the following.

1. Steroids, oral or topical.
2. Salicyates or other drugs with anti-prostaglandin effects.
3. Antihistamines.
4. Decongestants, oral and topical.
5. Hyposensitisation (allergy therapy).
6. Mucolytic agents: oral (Khan et al, 1981) or by injection into the middle ear cavity (Bauer, 1975).
7. Politzerisation.
8. Myringotomy.
9. Myringotomy with suction.
10. Insertion of ventilating tubes (grommets).
11. Adenoidectomy.
12. Mastoidectomy.

Of these measures, myringotomy with insertion of grommets (Fig. 4.10) produces the most immediate improvement in hearing. However the studies of Sadé (1979) underline that this benefit is only temporary. After 6–12 months there is no significant difference between the hearing of children who have been left untreated, have

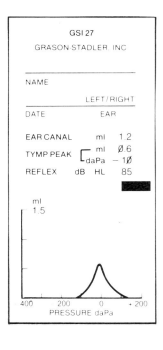
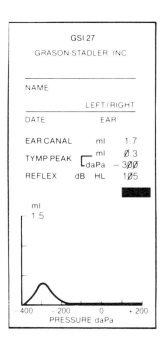

(a) (b)

Fig. 4.9. (a) Normal tympanogram: normal ear canal volume, normal middle ear mobility, normal middle ear pressure, normal reflex
(b) Poorly functioning Eustachian tube: normal ear canal volume, restricted mobility, abnormal middle ear pressure, reflex – slightly elevated. Possible cause: poorly functioning Eustachian tube, possibly some fluid

MIDDLE EAR DISORDERS 47

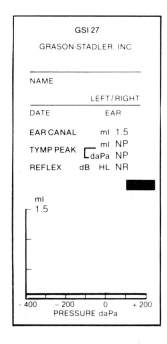
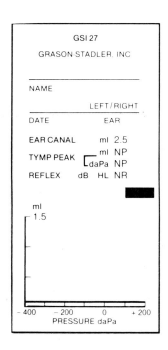

(c) (d)

(c) Serious otitis media: normal ear canal volume, no mobility, no middle ear pressure, no reflex. Possible cause: fluid filled middle ear (serious otitis media). Compliance peak may be present at a much more negative pressure than −400 daPa
(d) Tympanic membrane perforation: abnormal ear canal volume, no mobility, no middle ear pressure, no reflex. Possible cause: open perforation. Patent pressure equalisation (P–E) tube

48 EAR, NOSE AND THROAT DISORDERS

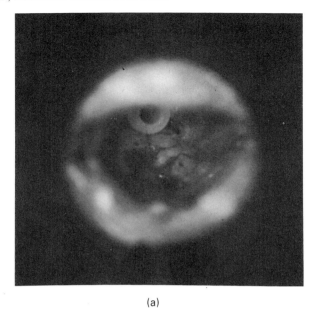

(a)

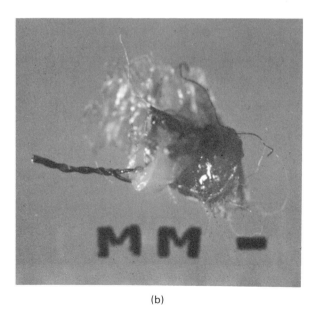

(b)

Fig. 4.10. (a) Grommet in situ. (b) Extruded grommet (courtesy of Mr Alan Fuller)

merely had a grommet inserted, have had a grommet plus aspiration of glue, or have had aspiration of glue, a grommet inserted, and adenoidectomy.

It has to be decided therefore whether the benefits of temporary hearing gain outweigh the risks and disadvantages of surgery in each individual case.

A major disadvantage of grommets for children has been debarrment from swimming. However of 100 children encouraged to swim with their grommets only three had any subsequent trouble (Jaffee, 1981). These developed otorrhoea, which cleared up with ear drops or oral penicillin and they returned to swimming with no further trouble. All the children had been instructed to put three drops of Neomycin/Polymixin/Hydrocortistone solution (as in Otosporin-Calmic) in the ear at bedtime each day they had been swimming. None used ear plugs or bathing caps. From this evidence it would seem unnecessary to deny swimming to children with grommets.

The efficacy of decongestant/antihistamine mixtures in glue ear remains controversial. The most recently reported, largest, and best constructed study (Cantekin et al, 1983) confirmed that treatment with a decongestant/antihistamine mixture cannot be expected to rid the middle ear of glue within 1 month (the duration of the trial). This has been a common observation in general practice. There is no evidence to deny the value of much longer courses of decongestant/antihistamine mixtures in promoting the clearing of middle ear fluid, nor in discouraging reaccumulation. Mucolytic agents such as S-carboxymethylcysteine (Mucodyne, Mucolex) have been reported to promote resolution of middle ear effusion (Hughes, 1983; Khan, 1983) and proposed as an alternative to surgery (Khan et al, 1981).

Management plan in general practice

Currently, a reasonable policy for glue ear in general practice would appear to be as follows.

a. Where hearing loss is not severe, for example less than 30 dB at speech frequencies, the upper respiratory tract should be rendered as healthy as possible, with antibiotics (usually Penicillin-V) where indicated. A decongestant/antihistamine mixture (such as Dimotapp Elixir) should be prescribed. A mucolytic agent should also be considered. Arrangements should be made for the child to sit near the front of the class at school. Regular observation should be made every 1 or 2 months.

b. If hearing loss is over 30 dB and remains so for more than 2 or 3 months despite medical treatment, the child should be referred for myringotomy, and probably insertion of grommets.

The interested general practitioner with access to an audiometer is in an ideal position to supervise the management of children not requiring surgery.

For best results it is important that general practitioner and specialist should agree a management policy, and know each other well enough to co-operate closely.

CHRONIC SUPPURATIVE OTITIS MEDIA

Introduction

Active chronic suppurative otitis media (CSOM) is characterised by t.m. perforation, otorrhoea, and deafness. There are two broad types of CSOM (Fig. 4.11).

1. 'Tubo-tympanic', in which the perforation is central and discharge, when present, tends to be copious, mucoid or mucopurulent. The perforation may vary in size from a pin-hole to a large kidney shaped 'sub-total' defect. Tubo-tympanic CSOM is often called 'safe' since it generally represents an inconvenience to the patient rather than a serious threat to health. Previous infection (perhaps inadequately treated) appears to play an important role in aetiology. Repeated t.m. perforation during attacks of otitis media damages the t.m. beyond recovery, resulting in a permanent defect. The existence of an established perforation predisposes to repeated re-infection of the middle ear from air-borne organisms.

2. Attico-antral CSOM is characterised by a marginal perforation, involving either the membrana flaccida in the attic region or the upper posterior rim of the t.m. The perforation is usually small, and the discharge thick, scanty, and evil smelling. The perforation may be concealed by debris, crusting, granulations or a polyp, and difficult to see. Attico-antral CSOM is associated with cholesteatoma formation. Negative middle ear pressure resulting from inadequate Eustachian ventilation (likely to have caused persistent glue ear in childhood) leads to invagination of the t.m. at the pars flaccida or at a site weakened by previous perforation. Negative pressure tends to be greatest in this region of the middle ear since

MIDDLE EAR DISORDERS 51

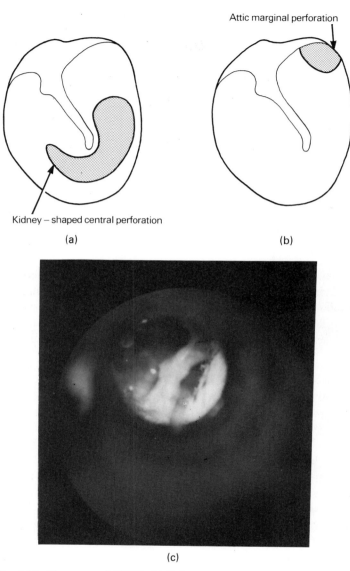

Fig. 4.11. Two types of CSOM. (a) Tubo-tympanic CSOM. (b) Attico-antral CSOM. (c) Tubo-tympanic CSOM.

it is furthest from the Eustachian tube and likely to be 'sealed off' by disease further forward. The squamous epithelium of the invaginated sac continues to grow, resulting in an accumulation of keratin: 'cholesteotoma' (Fig. 4.12).

52 EAR, NOSE AND THROAT DISORDERS

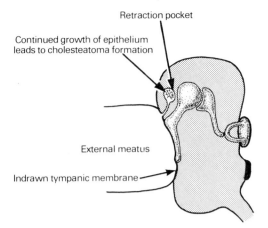

Fig. 4.12. Invaginated attic region leading to cholesteatoma

Because of its association with cholesteatoma, attico-antral CSOM is dangerous (Fig. 4.13). Expanding cholesteatomas may erode bone, increasing deafness by destruction of ossicles, and producing labyrinthitis from fistula formation especially into the horizontal semicircular canal or oval or round windows. Facial palsy

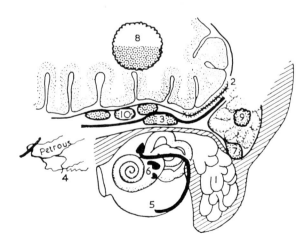

Key: 1. Mastoiditis. 2. Meningitis. 3. Extradural abscess. 4. Petrositis. 5. Facial nerve paralysis. 6. Labyrinthitis. 7. Lateral sinus thrombosis. 8. Temporal lobe abscess. 9. Cerebellar abscess. 10. Subdural abscess.

Fig. 4.13. Complications of middle ear infection (courtesy of Mr Miles Foxen and Blackwell Scientific Publication).

results from erosion into the facial canal. Mastoiditis is a common complication. Further bone destruction, opening the way for infection, may lead to extradural abscess, lateral sinus thrombosis, meningitis, temporal lobe or cerebellar abscess, – or by extension into the apex of the petrous temporal bone may give rise to Gradenigo's syndrome (p. 39).

Whilst most cases of cholesteatoma result from invagination of squamous epithelium as 'retraction pockets', squamous epithelium may also 'invade' the middle ear through a perforation, or may rarely result from embryological epithelial 'rests': congenital cholesteatoma.

The designation of tubo-tympanic CSOM as 'safe' is not entirely reliable. In a series of 202 consecutive cases of cholesteatoma operated upon in a 15-year period, Gristwood (1981, pers comm) encountered a central perforation in over 20%, and in 6.5% the t.m. was intact.

Presentation

Discharge is the commonest presenting symptom. Some degree of deafness is always present, but some patients are unaware of this until it is drawn to their attention. Discomfort in the ear is common, but more severe pain is uncharacteristic, and suggests either an episode of acute infection or the onset of dangerous complications.

Otitis externa is often present, secondary to the presence of middle ear discharge – and may mask the underlying middle ear disease unless the t.m. is inspected carefully and repeatedly.

Clinical course

The state of the ear in CSOM at any stage represents a balance between forces of destruction and repair.

Tubo-tympanic CSOM in children tends to run a benign course. With a declining propensity for upper respiratory tract infections as adolescence approaches, many small perforations heal spontaneously and hearing loss is often only slight. Long established perforations in adults are unlikely to heal spontaneously unless very small. Apart from the risk of acute otitis media if water enters the ear (for example through swimming or ill-advised syringing) the presence of a dry central perforation may cause little inconvenience, and if the perforation is small and anteriorly placed hearing loss may be minimal. More posteriorly placed central perforations expose the round window and interfere more with the 'ventilation' of sound waves through it (p. 69).

In attico-antral CSOM the disease process may remain quiescent for months, years, or even decades. At any stage however, insidious bone erosion may lay open a route for infection to invade the inner ear or contents of the middle or posterior cranial fossae.

The development of pain in patients who have had quiescent CSOM for many years is ominous and calls for full investigation.

Investigation

Patients with CSOM are likely to have an external meatus full of mucopus when first seen – this should be swabbed for bacteriology and sensitivites, then mopped away with cotton wool pledgets mounted on a Jobson-Horne probe.

Inspection of the t.m. for perforations is greatly facilitated if an inflation bulb is attached to the electric auriscope, or if a Seigle's speculum is used. Retraction pockets can then be distinguished from perforations, and mucopus may be seen oozing from a perforation as suction is applied.

Central perforations are easily seen, but defects in the attic or postero-superior marginal region are sometimes obscure, hidden beneath small crusts or debris. A characteristic evil smell is virtually pathognemonic of cholesteatoma.

The fistula sign should be sought – pressure on the tragus to compress air in the middle ear results in increased pressure in the labyrinth, with momentary giddiness, if bone erosion has created a communication between middle and inner ears.

An audiogram should be recorded to document the current state of hearing.

Management of CSOM in general practice

Tubo-tympanic CSOM

For patients with inactive tubo-tympanic CSOM, and a dry perforation, surgery to close the perforation (myringoplasty, or if ossicular damage is present, tympanoplasty) should be considered. This will close a potential route for re-infection of the middle ear, and may result in improved hearing. Patients willing to consider surgery will be referred to an ENT surgeon. Some, however, have no desire to swim, are no longer prone to ear infections, and have such minimal hearing loss that they are unwilling to contemplate surgery. Care of these cases is well within the scope of general practice: periodical inspection to keep the ear clean by dry mopping is the chief requisite. Since some hearing loss is inevitable it is important to avoid super-added deafness from wax accumulation.

Where active infection is present, regular toilet with instillation of antibiotic/steroid drops will often result in resolution and a 'dry' ear. Antibiotics are also effective orally. Reports on bacteriological swabs may lead to revision of choice of antibiotic. Even if the patient is to be referred to an ENT out-patient department, steps by the general practitioner to combat infection are helpful especially if the appointment is delayed.

Children with perforated ear drums. These present a special problem. Surgical closure with an underlay graft (myringoplasty) should be advised once the child has outgrown the tendency to repeated upper respiratory infection: there is a serious risk of break-down of the graft if further acute otitis media occurs. Operation is therefore usually delayed until the age of 10 or 11 years. In the meantime the ear must be kept dry. Mucoid discharge should be removed by frequent mopping with cotton wool pledgets twisted on a matchstick, a procedure which can be taught to the mother or older patient. Where discharge is purulent, antibiotics by mouth and/or topically (chloramphenicol/steroid mixtures such as 'Otopred' are suitable) are indicated.

Attico-antral CSOM

All cases of attico-antral disease should be referred for full ENT work-up. This will normally include examination under the microscope, and mastoid X-rays, in order to establish the extent of the disease and plan further management. Occasionally attico-antral CSOM is sufficiently quiescent for a provisional policy of regular follow-up alone to be adequate.

Surgery

In many cases of attico-antral CSOM surgery will be required to determine the extent of the disease.

Atticotomy. This alone may suffice: the middle ear is entered by a transmeatal approach and the t.m. reflected forwards. All cholesteatoma is removed and it may be necessary to sacrifice infected portions of the ossicles. If the surgeon is confident that all disease has been removed he may replace the t.m., with a graft if necessary. Otherwise a defect is left in the attic region to allow drainage and to facilitate subsequent microscopic examination and cleaning.

Attico-antrostomy, in which the mastoid antrum is also opened, is required where disease is more extensive.

Mastoidectomy, via a post-aural approach is called for with more extensive disease. In the operation of *radical mastoidectomy* the t.m., ossicles and mastoid air cells are all removed. The posterior meatal wall is removed down to the level of the facial canal creating one large cavity.

Sometimes a *modified radical mastoidectomy* is feasible, preserving some of the ossicles and t.m. This is designed to conserve as much hearing as possible, and has the added advantage that the ear should subsequently be dry since the Eustachian tube is 'closed off' from the mastoid cavity (Fig. 4.14).

Combined approach tympanoplasty. This is an operation which gained favour during the 1960s. The objective was, by means of both transmeatal and postaural approaches, to remove all cholesteatoma, and restore the integrity of the middle ear. The ossicular chain was reconstructed, often using a plastic prosthesis. The posterior wall of of the external meatus was preserved. It was hoped to leave the patient with good hearing and no mastoid cavity. Unfortunately it has proved impossible in most cases to remove all disease, and most patients have subsequently developed recurrence of cholesteatoma necessitating a radical mastoid operation. Enthusiasm for the operation has ceased in most centres. Those patients in whom further surgery has not yet been carried out must be assiduously followed up as most will probably eventually develop recurrent cholesteatoma.

After-care of mastoid cavities

Patients who have undergone radical mastoidectomy are normally followed up indefinitely in the ENT out-patient department. The cavities, if neglected, are liable to become filled with wax and debris which may become difficult and distressing to remove and may lead to ulceration, infection, and pain. Sometimes follow-up arrangements break down, for example if the patient moves to a new district. Fresh out-patient review may be arranged locally, but supervision of most mastoid cavities is well within the scope of the

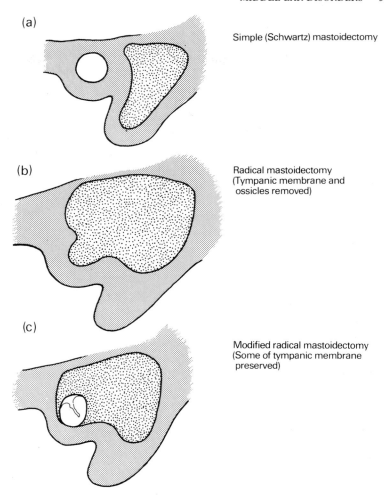

Fig. 4.14. (a) Simple (Schwartze) mastoidectomy. (b) Radical mastoidectomy (tympanic membrane and ossicles removed). (c) Modified radical mastoidectomy (some of tympanic membrane preserved).

interested general practitioner. Three-monthly, six-monthly, or annual inspection normally suffices. The mastoid 'bowl' is examined through a large speculum and wax and debris gently cleared using a wax hook or Jobson Horne probe. If the cavity epithelium appears moist or infected, insufflation of a little power (for example Cicatrin puffed from an original pack) is helpful.

Pschological aspects of CSOM

CSOM is in many ways a difficult and unsatisfactory condition to manage. Even in the best hands a small proportion (some 2%) of children have inadequate Eustachian tube function and proceed inexorably through glue ear problems, attacks of otitis media, discharging ears, countless ENT out-patients appointments, removal of tonsils and adenoids, and increasingly aggresive procedures leading finally to radical mastoidectomy. Even this may not be the end of the patient's troubles. The mastoid cavity may never become epithelialised with healthy skin, and may continue to discharge, despite the best endeavours, for years. Further surgery with revision of the mastoid cavity and excision of pockets of disease may be required. The disease is often bilateral, giving rise to serious deafness. It is often difficult to supply a satisfactory hearing aid insert in the presence of a mastoid cavity, and the wearing of a hearing aid is extremely unsatisfactory in the presence of discharge.

Patients who have undergone radical mastoidectomy, entailing removal of the t.m., are left with a communication from the postnasal space via the Eustachian tube to the outside through the ear. A resultant discharge of mucoid material from the ear may set up troublesome otitis externa. If the implications of loss of the t.m. have not been explained before the radical mastoidectomy operation, patients are liable to conclude that disease has returned and that their operation has been yet another failure.

CSOM patients often have an unhappy lot, and may become rather bitter, depressed, and disenchanted with medical care.

For the surgeon CSOM may pose a thankless dilemma. There is still no satisfactory surgical technique available to correct Eustachian tube obstruction, probably the fundamental cause of CSOM. All the surgeon can hope to do is to ameliorate its consequences. In his choice of surgical procedures he may be torn between the conflicting policies of conservatism, in order to preserve as much hearing as possible, and a more radical approach to ensure removal of all disease.

The patient who eventually comes to radical mastoidectomy may wonder why his operation was not performed much sooner. The co-operation of patients with CSOM may forgivably flag at times, and the support of an understanding general practitioner can be invaluable.

TRAUMA

Traumatic rupture of the tympanic membrane

The t.m. may be ruptured by penetration of a foreign body, by severe barotrauma, by sudden pressure change (as may result from a blow on the ear or explosive blast), and may complicate fracture of the skull.

Deafness and tinnitus are the chief symptoms: continuing pain is uncommon.

Treatment

Treatment is essentially to leave well alone. Spontaneous healing with full recovery of hearing is almost invariable. Rarely, the onset of infection may call for systemic antibiotics, and early surgical repair has been advocated where gross disruption of the drum has occurred (resulting from some blast injuries).

Otitic barotrauma

This term is applied to injury of the middle ear resulting from increase in atmospheric pressure, usually from descent in an aircraft or when diving underwater. It occurs when Eustachian tube function is inadequate to permit equalisation of pressures on either side of the t.m.

During ascent there is no problem – air escapes easily [Fig. 4.15(a)] whether or not the Eustachian tube is opened by muscular action. On decent, air must travel in the opposite direction, up the Eustachian tube to the middle ear cavity to allow pressure equalisation. The naso-pharyngeal end of the Eustachian tube can act almost like a one-way valve. Entry of air in a 'retrograde' direction requires active opening of the orifice by muscular contraction. Once sufficient pressure differential has built up between the nasopharynx and the tube lumen, muscular contraction may be inadequate to open the orifice; the tube is 'locked' [Fig. 4.15(b)]. As descent continues the t.m. becomes forced increasingly inwards by rising exterior pressure. It becomes wrapped around the middle ear structures. The extreme negative pressure within the middle ear cavity leads to oedema, and echymoses of the mucous membrane, and often a bloody transudate. Finally, the t.m. may rupture.

60 EAR, NOSE AND THROAT DISORDERS

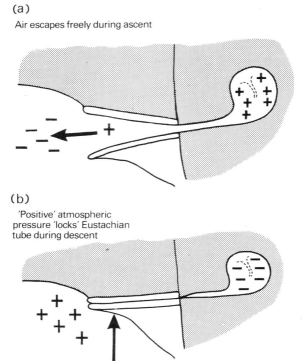

Fig. 4.15. Mechanism of barotrauma: Eustachian tube function. (a) Air escapes freely during ascent. (b) 'Positive' atmospheric pressure 'locks' Eustachian tube during descent.

The condition is often extremely painful, and leads to deafness, tinnitus, and occasional vertigo. Patients often complain of a sensation of 'fluid in the ear'. On inspection the t.m. is typically reddened and dull. It is likely to be indrawn, bubbles are occasionally discernable in the middle ear, and occasionally the t.m. is ruptured.

Treatment

Most cases resolve spontaneously. Decongestant nasal drops and decongestant oral preparations such as Dimotapp should promote recovery. Antibiotics are indicated if there is any suspicion of infection (sometimes the condition appears to have arisen as a consequence of flying with an upper respiratory infection).

Where symptoms are severe, immediate relief is provided by

myringotomy. It is often thought desirable at this stage to insert a grommet to ensure good middle ear ventilation until recovery is complete.

Persons subject to otitic barotrauma when flying should make use of decongestants half an hour before descent is due, and should remain awake during descent, and carry out frequent Valsalva manoeuvres.

REFERENCES

Bain D J G 1981 Acute otitis media in general practice. The Practitioner 225:1568
Bauer F 1975 Tubal function in glue ear: urea for glue ears. Journal of Laryngology and Otology 89 (1):63
Biedel C W 1978 American Journal of Diseases of Childhood 132: 681–683
Branefors-Hedlander P, Dahlberg T, Ny Len O 1975 Acute otitis media – frequent episodes. Acta Otolaryngolica. 80: 399–409
Brooks D N 1976 School screening for middle ear effusions. Annals of Otology, Rhinology & Laryngology 85 (suppl 25):223
Cantekin E I, Mandel E M, Bluestone C D, Rockette H E, Paradise J L, Stool S E, Fria T J, Rogers K D 1983 Lack of efficacy of a decongestant/antihistamine combination for otitis media with effusion ('secretory' otitis media) in children. New England Journal of Medicine 308(6): 297–301
Fry J 1972 Acute otitis media, International Handbook of Medical Science 2nd edn. Medical & Technical Publishing Co Ltd, Oxford. p 627–629
Gristwood R E 1981 Personal communication
Hallett C P 1982 Re screening and epidemiology of middle ear disease in a population of primary school infants. Journal of Laryngology and Otology 96: 899–914
Hibbert J, Stell P M 1982 The role of enlarged adenoids in the aetiology of serous otitis media. Clinical Otolaryngology 7: 253–256
Hoffman-Lawless K, Keith R W, Cotton R T 1981 Auditory processing in children with previous middle ear effusion. Annals of Otolaryngology 90: 543–545
Hughes K B 1983 A comparative study of mucodyne and a decongestant combination in otitis media with effusion. Royal Society of Medicine Forum Series (5) Mucoregulation in Respiratory Tract Disorders pages 23–25 (Published by the Royal Society of Meduine London)
Jaffee B F 1981 Are water and tympanotomy tubes compatible?. The Laryngoscope 91 (4):563
Jordan R 1949 Chronic secretory otitis media. Laryngoscope 59:1002
Juhn S K 1982 Studies on middle ear effusions. Laryngoscope 92: 287–291
Khan J A 1983 A comparative study of mucodyne and a decongestant combination in otitis media with effusion. Royal Society of Medicine Forum Series (5) Mucorequlation in Respiratory Tract Disorders pages 19–22 (Published by the Royal Society of Medicine London)
Khan J A, Kirkwood E M, Lewis C 1981 Immunological aspects of secretory otitis media in children. 1gE & 1gA levels in serum & glue. Journal of Laryngology and Otology 95: 121–123
Khan J A, Marcuss P, Cummings S W 1981 S-carboxymethylcysterine in otitis media with effusion. Journal of Laryngology and Otology 95: 995–1001

Klein J O, Teele D W 1976 Isolation of viruses and mycoplasms from middle ear effusions. A review. Annals of Otology, Rhinology & Laryngology 85 (Suppl 25): 140–144

Makela P H, Karma P 1981 Pneumococcal vaccine in otitis media. Lancet i:152

Marks N J, Mills R P, Shaheen O H 1981 A controlled trial of cotrimoxazole therapy in serous otitis media. Journal of Laryngology and Otology 95: 1003–1009

Maw A R, Jeans W D, Cable H R 1983 Adenoidectomy. A prospective study to show clinical and radiological changes 2 years after operation. Journal of Laryngology and Otology 97: 511–518

Mawson S R, Brennand J 1969 Longterm follow up of 129 glue ears. Proceedings of the Royal Society of Medicine 62: 460–463

Paradise J L 1981 Antimicrobial prophylaxis for recurrent otitis media. Annals of Otology. Rhinology and Laryngology 90 (Suppl 84):56

Research conference on recent advances in otitis media with effusion 1980 Report. Annals of Otolaryngology May–June (Suppl 69)3: 19–21

Sadé J 1979 In: Secretory otitis media and its sequelae. Churchill Livingstone, London 269

Schutte P K, Beales D L, Dalton R 1981 Secretory otitis media, a retrospective study. Journal of Laryngology and Otology 95: 17–22

Schwartz R, Rodriguez J, Khan W N, Ross S 1977. Acute purulent otitis media in children older than 5 years. Journal of the American Medical Association 238:1032

Schwartz R H, Rodriguez W J, Schwartz D M 1981 Office myringotomy for acute otitis media: its value in preventing middle ear effusion. The Laryngoscope 91: 616–619

Shurin P A, Pelton S I, Donner A, Klein J O 1979 Persistence of middle ear effusion after acute otitis media in children. New England Journal of Medicine 300:1121

Tos M 1981 Upon the relationship between secretory otitis in childhood and chronic otitis and its sequale in adults. Journal of Laryngology and Otology 95: 1011–1022

Tos M, Holm – Jensen S, Sørensen C H, Mogensen C 1982 Spontaneous course and frequency of secretory otitis in 4 year old children. Archives of Otolaryngology 108: 4–10

Veltri R W, Sprinkle P M 1976 Secretory otitis media. An immune complex disease. Annals of Otology. Rhinology and Laryngology 85(Suppl 25):135

Wather J 1755 A method proposed to restore the hearing when injured from an obstruction of the tube Eustachiana. Physiological Transactions of the Royal Society of London (Biol Sci) 49:213

Wisbey A S 1983 Dyslexia. The Ophthalmic Optician Jan 1:10

5

Deafness

APPLIED ANATOMY OF INNER EAR. MECHANISM OF HEARING

The inner ear is essentially an elaborate compartmentalised intercommunicating sac [the *membranous* labyrinth, Fig. 5.1(a)] distended with endolymph and floating in perilymph within a series of chambers [the *bony* labyrinth, Fig. 5.1(b)] within the petrous temporal bone. It contains the sensory organs of hearing and balance at the ends of branches of the 8th nerve.

The bony labyrinth, visible in suitable skull X-rays, consists of three portions: the semicircular canals, the vestibule, and the cochlea. The oval and round windows perforate the lateral wall of the vestibule, providing functional communication with the middle ear cavity via the stapes footplate and secondary t.m. respectively.

The membranous labyrinth consists of the three membranous semicircular canals, the utricle and saccule in the bony vestibule, and the cochlear duct in the bony cochlea. The endolymph within differs chemically from the perilymph, having a higher potassium and lower sodium concentration.

The semicircular canals communicate with the utricle, and the utricle and saccule are connected by the Y shaped endolymphatic duct, the stem of which becomes the saccus endolymphaticus. The latter passes through a bony canal to end blindly close to, or in, the dura in the posterior cranial fossa. (Veins around the saccus drain directly into the sigmoid sinus and are believed to be concerned in endolymphatic absorption).

The saccule communicates with the cochlear duct via the ductus reuniens.

The sensory neuro-epithelium of the semicircular canals, utricle

64 EAR, NOSE AND THROAT DISORDERS

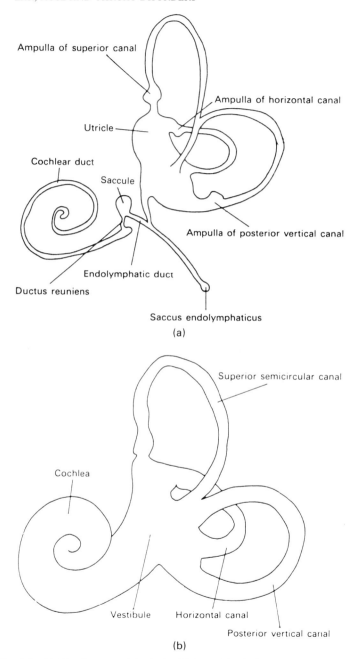

Fig. 5.1. (a) Membraneous labyrinth. (b) bony labyrinth.

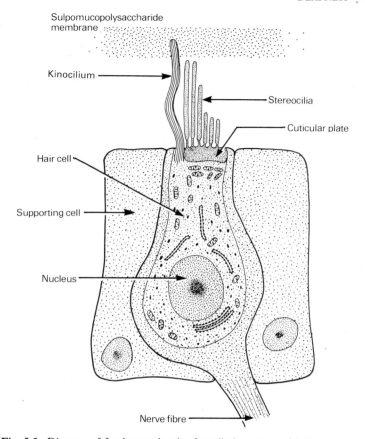

Fig. 5.2. Diagram of fundamental unit of vestibular neuro-epithelium.

and saccule, and cochlear duct possesses a broadly similar structure (Fig. 5.2) being composed essentially of hair-bearing cells, supporting cells, and an overlying jelly-like substance (sulphomucopolysaccharide) into which the hairs protrude.

Each semicircular canal has a dilatation (the ampulla, Fig. 5.3) containing a sensory area ('crista') which bears hair cells with overlying gelatinous material (here called the 'cupola'). Movement of endolymph within the canal causes distortion of the cupola, sensed by the hair-bearing cells and enabling appreciation of acceleration.

The utricle contains similar hair cells at a site, the macula, lying in an approximately horizontal plane. Calcite crystals (statoconia) are embedded in the overlying sulphomucopolysaccharide 'otolith

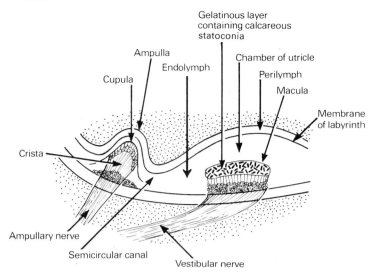

Fig. 5.3 Diagram of ampulla of semicircular canal and macula of utricle.

membrane', and pulled by gravity enable the hair cells to appreciate the position of the head in space.

The saccule bears a similar macula on its medial wall, in the vertical plane.

The cochlear duct (scala media) spirals 2.5 times within the bony cochlea. Containing endolymph, it is sandwiched between two spiral tubes containing perilymph (Figs. 5.4 & 5.5). The upper tube (scala vestibuli) is separated from the middle ear at the oval window by the stapes footplate, and is continuous at the apex of the cochlea (helicotrema) with the lower tube (scala tympani). The latter is separated from the middle ear at the round window by the secondary t.m. The scala tympani also communicates with the subarachnoid space via the cochlear aqueduct running in the cochlear canaliculus.

The cochlear duct is essentially triangular in cross section, the base being formed by the basilar membrane, stretching from the osseous spiral lamina at the centre of the cochlear spiral (modiolus) to the spiral ligament on the outer wall. The outer wall of the triangle is formed by the stria vascularis, and the hypotenuse by Reissner's membrane.

The organ of Corti, the sense organ of hearing, runs as a spiral on the basilar membrane, and like the organs of balance is composed of hair cells, supporting cells, and an overlying gelatinous material (here called the tectorial membrane). The hair cells are

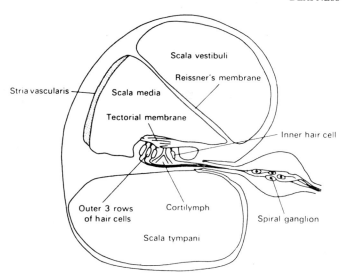

Fig. 5.4. Section through one turn of cochlea.

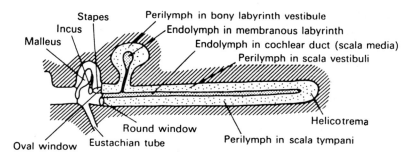

Fig. 5.5. Diagram of cochlea 'straightened out'.

arranged as an inner single row and an outer group three or four rows wide. Each ear contains about 4500 inner and 12 500 outer hair cells. Hairs (stereocilia) projecting into the tectorial membrane are attached to the cuticular membrane at the top of each hair cell. Cochlear microphonics are believed to be generated at the cuticular membrane.

A cross-section shows the inner and outer rows of hair cells to be separated by two 'pillars of Corti' which meet above to enclose a space – the tunnel of Corti, containing cortilymph. This appears to be continuous with the perilymph in the scala tympani: its significance is as yet unknown.

Innervation of the inner ear

Afferent fibres from the vestibular neuroepithelium, constituting the ampullary, utricular, and saccular nerves, unite to form the vestibular nerve and synapse in the vestibular ganglion in the internal auditory meatus.

Afferent fibres from the organ of Corti pass in the osseous spiral lamina towards the modiolus, and synapse in the spiral ganglion, whence a second relay of fibres coalesce to form the cochlear nerve. This runs alongside the vestibular nerve in the internal auditory meatus to reach the brain. Some of the first relay of afferent fibres come directly from inner hair cells, each fibre arising from several hair cells and each hair cell being innervated by several fibres. The remainder of the first relay of afferent fibres arise from outer hair cells, many running spirally for about one-third of the cochlea and communicating with many outer hair cells, and each hair cell communicating with many fibres, before turning towards the modiolus. In addition to these afferent fibres (some 25 000) there are about 500 efferent fibres passing from the brain to the hair cells.

Evidence is mounting that impulses conveyed in these fibres are associated with tinnitus.

Blood supply

The labyrinth is supplied by the labyrinthine artery. This usually arises from the anterior inferior cerebellar artery, a branch of the midline basilar artery. Occasionally it arises direct from the basilar artery or even from the vertebral artery. It travels in the internal auditory meatus and branches to supply the inner ear. The cochlear branch travels around the modiolus sending some branches out along the osseous spiral lamina and others upward over the 'roof' of the turn of the cochlea to supply the stria vascularis, – a network of capillaries composed of endothelium only, thought to be involved in formation and absorption of endolymph.

Mechanism of hearing

The pinna serves a limited but useful function in collecting sound and deflecting it into the external auditory meatus. Some reinforcement of entering sound vibrations is provided by the mechanical effect of the ratio between the length of the handle of the malleus and the long process of the incus: 1.3 to 1.0. Further increase in sound vibration force results from the ratio between the areas of the t.m. and oval window areas, estimated at 14 to 1. The combined effect of these ratios is to increase the force of sound vibrations by a factor of 18.3. Loss of this vibration enhancing capacity, as resulted from fenestration operations, frequently led to a 30 dB hearing loss; of the order to be expected on theoretical grounds.

Conduction of sound vibration to the organ of Corti is normally achieved by movement of the stapedial footplate piston within the oval window. Vibrations thus conveyed to the perilymph travel into the scala vestibuli, thence to the scala tympani via the helicotrema, and may then be thought of as being 'ventilated to the exterior' via the round window. Sandwiched between the scala vestibuli and scala tympani, the scala media, enclosing the organ of Corti, receives these vibrations. Without an intact t.m. and ossicular chain (the situation following a radical mastoidectomy operation) a hearing loss of 40–60 dB occurs. The magnitude of this loss is partly due to the fact that air vibrations reach the oval and round windows with equal force, and normal 'circulation' of sound in the inner ear is prevented.

Detection of sound signals and their conversion into action potentials in the auditory nerve is a function of the hair cells. The point along the basilar membrane at which the hair cells are stimulated by sound vibrations depends on the sound frequency. Microphonic potentials generated by stimulation of hair cells follow faithfully the wave form and amplitude of the acoustic stimulus.

Acoustic vibrations reaching the scala vestibuli induce in the basement membrane a so-called 'travelling wave' which begins at the basal end and moves toward the apex. The area of maximum displacement of the basilar membrane varies with the frequency. High pitched sounds produce a short travelling wave limited to the basal turn. Lower frequency stimuli give waves with maximum displacement progressively nearer the apex.

It is believed that high frequency sounds, above 5000 Hz, are perceived in the basal turn hair cells only, whilst low frequency sounds (below 400 Hz) are appreciated along the entire organ of Corti, and give rise to action potentials in the individual auditory nerve fibres which are synchronous with the stimulating sound. Intermediate frequencies are conveyed to the brain by groups of two, three or four fibres which 'fire' in succession, overcoming the limitation imposed by the refractory period of individual fibres at these frequencies. Appreciation of variations in loudness is thought to be mediated by variations in numbers of auditory fibres stimulated.

The outer row of hair cells appears to 'tune' the inner hair cells, causing their responsiveness to be highly frequency-specific at low source intensities. At higher sound intensities the inner hair cells respond to a widening band of neighbouring frequencies as well. The outer hair cells are particularly vulnerable to disease processes.

The auditory nerve afferent fibres end in the cochlear nucleus of the same side in the brain stem. Most of the next generation of fibres cross the midline and travel in the lateral lemniscus to the inferior colliculus or medial geniculate body. A further generation of fibres passes from the medial geniculate body to the higher auditory centres in the temporal lobe. Experiments with microelectrodes have shown that in the cochlear nucleus the cochlea is represented 'straightened out' and that some increase in sound resolution is achieved ('funnelling'): when a group of neurones in the cochlear nucleus is activated by sound of appropriate frequency, resting activity in surrounding neurones is inhibited.

Recruitment

A consequence of the vulnerability of the outer hair cells is the phenomenon of recruitment. This occurs in deafness of cochlear origin, where the outer hair cells have degenerated. The patient cannot hear quiet sounds, but suddenly becomes aware of noise as volume increases and the raised threshold of the untuned inner hair cells is reached. Thus a lorry approaching from behind is not heard until almost upon the patient, when the engine roar is suddenly heard with alarm. Similarly, the patient may not hear a quiet conversational voice, but when the voice is raised it is suddenly heard loudly, and the protest is provoked 'Don't shout! I'm not deaf!'.

DEAFNESS

Deafness is a common handicap. Recent figures from the Institute of Hearing Research in Nottingham indicate that some 10 000 000 people in Britain have a significant degree of hearing impairment. Between one and two babies/1000 are born with severe deafness which will subsequently require special educational measures. The incidence of deafness increases rapidly with advancing age: one-third of the adult population over 65 years has a hearing loss requiring an aid, yet only about one-half of this group admits to the problem and is issued with one. One-half of the population above the age of 80 years has a severe hearing loss.

Types of deafness

Deafness may be a. conductive, where the problem lies in the outer or middle ear, or b. sensorineural (also called 'perceptive') where the cause involves the cochlea ('cochlear' or 'sensory' deafness) or the 8th nerve and its central connections ('retrocochlear' or 'neural' deafness).

In many patients elements of both types of loss are present: 'mixed' deafness.

Conductive causes of deafness are often surgically remediable and, where this is not possible, a hearing aid gives good results.

Sensorineural deafness is beyond surgical help except in rare circumstances such as:
  a. perilymph fistula (p. 102)
  b. cochlear implant surgery – now being pioneered in several centres.

At present only the totally deaf can derive any benefit, and crude awareness of a tone is all that can be provided.

Recognition of deafness

Whilst most deaf patients seek help, some do not. They may be quite unaware of their handicap, or may regard it as being unimportant or a humiliation better ignored. Employability may be jeopardised. Such patients with unrecognised, unassisted deafness face unfortunate consequences. They fail to heed when spoken to, sometimes gaining an undeserved reputation for rudeness or even arrogance. Misunderstandings arise, implications for education are obvious, and road safety may be at risk. People with quite mild hearing losses also show apparent associated *memory* deficits (Rabbit, 1983, Personal communication).

By detecting and treating unrecognised deafness the general practitioner can render valuable service. Certain clues raise suspicion.

Hearing difficulty may be apparent as the patient is invited from the waiting room (he may stand up when someone with a similar name is called). Tell-tale signs in speech may be present: deaf people tend to mispronounce consonants, particularly 's'. They may appear to be looking at one's face with unduly close attention – lip reading.

Investigation of suspected deafness in the consulting room

The ear must first be inspected with an otoscope. Accumulations of wax can give a hearing loss of up to 20 dB, and must be removed before hearing can be assessed. The t.m. is examined.

A crude guide to hearing is obtained by asking the patient to repeat numbers, whispered first as quietly as possible, then spoken with increasing volume until heard. The examiner closes the patient's opposite ear with a finger on the tragus, and positions his mouth 1 m lateral to the test ear, out of the patient's field of vision. Very deaf people may only hear a shout close to the ear, and to ensure that he is not in fact hearing with the closed ear this may be 'masked' by noisily crumpling a piece of stiff paper close to that ear.

For young children, familiar words are used in testing instead of numbers.

Tuning fork tests

Where hearing is impaired, tuning fork tests serve to determine whether the fault is conductive or sensorineural. A tuning fork vibrating at 512 Hz is most commonly used. The doctor equipping himself for the first time is well advised to purchase a large, heavy fork [Fig. 5.6(b)]. Lighter forks are cheaper, but cease to vibrate relatively quickly after striking, leading to considerable confusion.

Rinne's test

The fork is struck and the base firmly applied to the patient's mastoid process. He is asked to lower his raised hand when he can no longer hear the sound. The fork is then transferred forwards and held so that the end of one prong is 1 cm from the ear, with the prongs in the same plane as the ear. If he can now hear the fork again the test is positive. If he cannot, the procedure is reversed. If the fork is heard longer by bone conduction the result is described as Rinne negative. A positive result is obtained in the normal ear and in sensorineural deafness. A negative result indicates conductive deafness.

A falsely negative Rinne's test may occur in cases of severe unilateral sensorineural deafness. No sound is heard by air conduction, but when bone conduction is tested sound is heard by conduction across the skull to the other ear. In such cases the better ear may

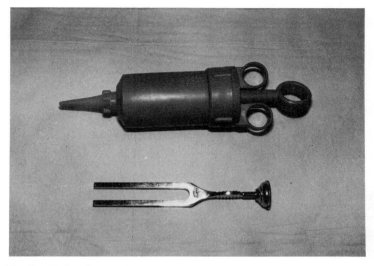

Fig. 5.6 (a) Shaw's ear syringe. (b) Tuning fork

be 'masked', for example by crumpling paper close to the ear, and the test repeated.

Weber's test

This test is useful where there is a marked difference in hearing on the two sides. The base of the vibrating fork is placed on the skull on the midline. Reference of the sound to the deaf ear indicates conductive deafness, whilst reference to the 'good' ear occurs in sensorineural deafness.

In order to explain reference to the deaf ear in conductive deafness it has been postulated that the conductive lesion excludes ambient noise, leaving the cochlea on that side free to 'concentrate' on the skull vibrations. The phenomenon however still occurs in a sound-proof room, and a more satisfactory explanation is probably that the conductive lesion preventing sound *entry* to the deaf ear also prevents sound *exit*.

A convenient way of recording the tuning fork findings in the notes is as follows.

$+ \overset{512}{\underset{\downarrow}{|}} +$ = Rinne positive on both sides. Weber not referred.
(As in normal hearing and in bilateral sensorineural deafness.)

74 EAR, NOSE AND THROAT DISORDERS

+(R)$\overset{512}{\swarrow}$ (L) + = Rinne positive (left). Positive (right).
Weber referred to right. (As in left sensorineural deafness.)

−(R)$\overset{512}{\swarrow}$ (L) + = Rinne negative (right). Positive (left).
Weber referred to right. (As in right conductive deafness.)

−(R) $\overset{512}{\updownarrow}$ (L) − = Rinne negative left and right.
Weber not referred.
(Indicates symmetrical conductive deafness.)

Audiometry

Whilst a pure-tone audiometer is not an essential part of a general practitioner's equipment, it greatly increases his effectiveness. Uses of audiometry in general practice include the following:

1. Monitoring of children with glue ear problems.
2. Identification of patients sufficiently deaf to require referral for trial of a hearing aid.
3. Surveillance of hearing in patients working in noisy conditions.
4. Follow-up of acute otitis media, mumps, and head injury where the suspicion of hearing difficulty exists.
5. Reassurance of over-anxious patients with minimal ear symptoms.
6. An audiometer is required for general practitioners approved to carry out such work as the routine examination of professional pilots and divers.
7. An audiometer should certainly be available in practices approved for general practice postgraduate training.

The simplest and cheapest audiometers are designed for screening, have a limited range (usually not above 4000 Hz), but serve most of the above functions adequately. More comprehensive portable audiometers (Fig. 5.7) have a wider range (250–8000 Hz), with facilities for bone conduction measurement and masking. The cost of such machines is approximately one-half that of an ECG machine.

The recording of a basic air conduction audiogram is simple and quick in most cases, taking less time than an electrocardiogram. The task is eminently suitable for a properly instructed practice nurse.

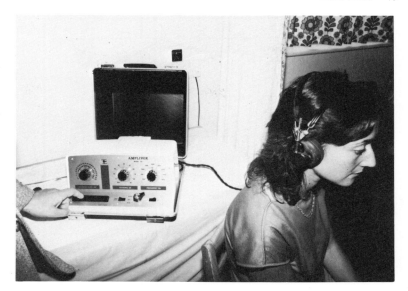

Fig. 5.7. Amplivox portable audiometer in use.

Method

A reasonably quiet room is needed for audiometry. The patient should be positioned so that he cannot see the operator's hands. He puts on the headphones, and is asked to raise his hand whenever he hears a sound (children may be given a more interesting task such as to transfer a marble from one box to another).

At each frequency, tones are presented to the test ear, and repeated at reduced volume, descending in 10 dB steps until no longer heard. Volume is then increased by 5 dB steps until the tone is just heard again. This volume is the threshold of the ear for the frequency in question.

It is customary to begin by testing hearing at 2000 Hz, then to work upwards and downwards to the limit of the audiometer. The results are plotted on a chart (Fig. 5.8) (by international agreement the symbol X is used to represent the left ear, and O for the right).

Where a hearing difference of more than 40 dB exists between the two ears, the possibility arises that loud tones apparently heard by the deafer ear are really heard by the better ear after travelling across the skull. To exclude this possibility it is necessary to 'mask' the better ear with 'white sound' delivered at volume 15 dB greater than the test tone. Simple screening audiometers do not have this facility, but it is provided on standard portable audiometers.

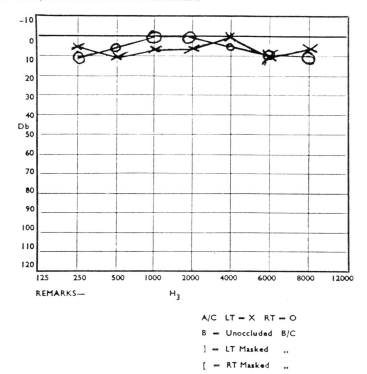

Fig. 5.8. Normal audiogram.

Where a hearing loss is demonstrated, its type – conductive, sensorineural, or mixed – is ascertained by measurement of bone conduction. A headband bearing a bone conduction headphone is placed so that the latter is pressed against the mastoid process. The ear on this side is uncovered by moving the air conduction headphone forward, and masking is delivered to the non-test ear through the headphone covering it. Hearing for sounds presented via the bone conductor is measured using the same procedure as for air conduction, and recorded using the symbols] for left ear bone conduction and [for right.

Other types of audiometry

Impedence audiometry

This is discussed on page 43.

Békésy audiometry

This is used primarily to screen patients at risk in noisy occupations. The patient presses a button on hearing test sounds presented by the machine automatically. In effect he writes his own audiogram.

Audiometry in special centres

More sophisticated audiometry in special centres is required for the following reasons.
1. To establish whether sensorineural deafness is 'cochlear' or 'retrocochlear'.
2. To measure hearing objectively in patients unable to cooperate (e.g. in the very young or mentally handicapped).
3. To identify 'non-organic' hearing loss.

Electric (evoked) response audiometry

In the last decade electric response audiometry has become available in major centres. Two types are in general use.
1. Transtympanic electrocochleography (Fig. 5.9(a)). A fine needle electrode is passed through the t.m. to lie against the promontary. Electric responses initiated in the cochlea and 8th nerve by sound signals are recorded. The method identifies thresholds, and gives information regarding disorders of inner ear function, particularly Menière's disease.
2. Brain-stem electric response audiometry (Fig. 5.9(b) & (c)). Electrodes are placed on the vertex of the skull and mastoid processes. Following a sound signal, seven waves may be distinguished during the first 10 ms. The first (N_1) is the 8th nerve action potential, N_2 arises from the cochlear nucleus, N_3 from the superior olive, N_4 from the nuclei of the lateral lemniscus, N_5 from the inferior colliculus, and N_6 and N_7 from higher in the auditory pathway.

This non-invasive objective method is invaluable for threshold testing in infants, young children, and suspected malingerers, in the diagnosis of acoustic neuromas, and in the diagnosis of brain-stem lesions including multiple sclerosis.

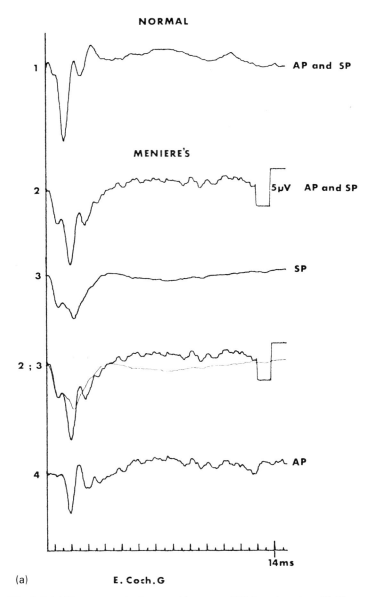

Fig. 5.9 (a) Transtympanic electrocochleograms: (1) Normal tracing; (2) Abnormal electrocochleogram in Menière's disease showing broadening of wave response due to summating potential (SP) from displaced basilar membrane (AP = action potential).

(b) Sites of origin of brain-stem auditory evoked response waves: I 8th nerve; II cochlear nucleus; III superior olive; IV lateral lemniscus. V inferior colliculus.

(c) Brain-stem evoked responses in a patient with a left acoustic neuroma. The delay in transmission of wave V caused by the tumour is evident on comparision with the right (normal) side.

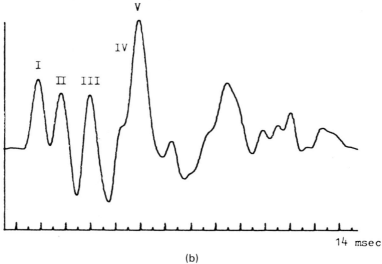

Fig. 5.9 a, b, c Courtesy of Dr Richard Billings, Dept. of Neurosciences, St Bartholomew's Hospital.

DEAFNESS IN INFANCY

Aquisition of language is fundamental to human development. In the second half of the first year the infant begins to 'babble' and gradually comes to imitate his mother's speech meaningfully. Before the end of the first year verbal communication is beginning, and during the second year vocabulary expands rapidly. Recognition of language in a visual form follows, and during the third year most children are beginning to hold conversations and to recognise written words. Many children are reading simple sentences by the age of 5 years.

This aquisition of language is intimately related to development in other spheres: physical, visual, locomotor, intellectual, and emotional.

Importance of early recognition

The deaf infant faces an enormous handicap in life, for if he is unable to hear his mother's speech the whole process of language aquisition and subsequent general development will fail. Most infants with a severe hearing loss nevertheless have 'islands' of hearing which are capable of exploitation with hearing-aids, enabling them to start on the developmental path at a more or less normal time. The rewards from the resulting change in the infant's prospects are incalculable.

It is therefore critically important that deafness in infants be identified at the earliest possible time, preferably before the age of 8 months, and certainly during the first 2 years of life. If deafness is missed until a later stage, the greatest opportunity for helping the child will have been lost.

A recent survey, by the National Deaf Children's Society, of 635 deaf children, revealed an average delay of nearly 2 years between parents first suspecting the child to be deaf and the diagnosis of deafness and provision of hearing aids. 41 per cent were not detected at their first screening even though by that time most parents thought their child had a hearing loss.

Causes of deafness in infancy

Certain infants are 'at risk' by reason of such factors as follows.

1. Heredity.

2. Infections during pregnancy, especially rubella, cytomegalovirus, syphilis and toxoplasmosis. The coils of the cochlea are already well formed by 6 weeks from conception.
3. Hyperbilirubinaemia. Rhesus incompatibility has been the major cause and this should now be eliminated by anti D vaccine.
4. Anoxia and toxaemia during pregnancy.
5. Prematurity.
6. Teratogenic drugs.
7. Congenital deformities resulting in malformations of the ear, and maxillofacial anomalies.
8. Birth injuries during difficult deliveries.
9. Meningitis in early infancy, especially from *Haemophilus influenzae* (Hof, 1976).

Table 5.1 shows the causes of sensorineural hearing loss in a group of 63 children seen in Manchester between 1975 and 1979 (Taylor, 1980).

Table 5.1

	Rubella	Cytomegalovirus	Meningitis	Birth history	Unknown	Other
Number	19	7	4	12	19	2
Percentage	30	11	6	19	30	4

That rubella was the cause of deafness in 30% is deplorable since it is entirely preventable. The National Congenital Rubella Programme reports an average of 67 children born each year with congenital rubella. Nowadays deafness is more likely to be the sole resulting handicap, presumably a consequence of the practice of termination in early pregnancy for maternal rubella. Rubella acquired later in pregnancy is likely to affect the ear alone, whilst in earlier pregnancy the heart, eyes, and brain are frequently affected as well.

In some 30% of children born with sensorineural deafness, the cause is unknown (recessive inheritance is thought to be chiefly responsible).

Prevention of deafness in infancy

The general practitioner's role is crucial, particularly since rubella is the single most preventable cause of congenital deafness. From the practice age/sex register it is possible to identify all women of childbearing age and where appropriate, to arrange a rubella antibody titre estimation. In the absence of adequate immunity, rubella vaccine can be administered under a 3-month contraception cover, and development of protective immunity confirmed by repeat antibody titre estimation.

Reliance upon a history of rubella or schoolgirl immunisation is unsatisfactory. Several viruses can give rise to an illness easily mistaken for rubella. Batches of vaccine are sometimes 'dud' and vaccine response in schoolgirls is not confirmed. Some schoolgirls are inevitably missed during immunisation sessions.

Increasing use of microcomputers in general practice should ease the task of identification and 'calling in' of appropriate women for antibody titre estimation – otherwise time consuming and expensive. In the absence of such a planned campaign, the opportunity should at least be taken to check the rubella antibody status of all eligible women attending the surgery, including all who come for contraceptive advice.

Problems associated with birth accounted for deafness in about one-fifth of the Manchester children. The general practitioner can often help by ensuring that high risk mothers are confined in departments where adequate expertise and special care baby units are available.

Meningitis in infancy is an important cause of sensorineural deafness. The general practitioner's high index of suspicion in any unwell infant is vital to ensure early treatment.

Recognition of deafness in infancy

Mothers (or grandmothers) of deaf children often begin to suspect something is amiss by the third month, and the greatest significance should be attached to their fears. The only way the matter can be satisfactorily settled may be by referral to a major ENT centre where brain-stem electric response audiometry is available. The sooner the true position is ascertained, and amplification and the services of a special children's hearing clinic obtained where necessary the better.

Screening

Ideally the hearing of all infants should be screened at birth using brain-stem electric response audiometry. This is impracticable: the cost of the equipment and scarcity of technicians would in any case be prohibitive. More promising is the 'Linco-Bennett' auditory response cradle (Fig. 5.10) based on the principal that if an infant moves, or his respiratory rate slows, with sufficient consistency within 2.5 s of a signal repeated many times good hearing is confirmed. The baby lies in the auditory response cradle, signals are emitted, and the infant's movements in response to these signals are sensed and recorded automatically. The current cost of the cradle is between £8000 and £9000.

Routine screening of children's hearing is a commitment of health visitors engaged by district health authorities. Increasingly, general practitioners are organising child development surveillance within their practices, in association with 'attached' health visitors.

Infant hearing testing should be performed when the infant is between 6 and 8 months old, and requires the co-operation of an assistant who endeavours to attract the infant's attention. The in-

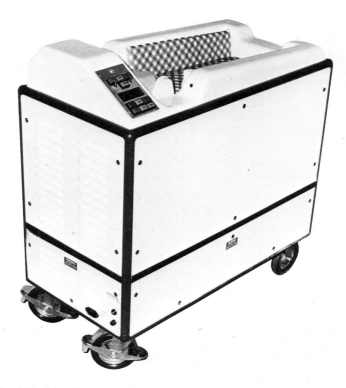

Fig. 5.10. Linco-Bennett auditory response cradle.

fant sits on his/her mother's knee and the tester, approaching from behind, makes low and high pitched sounds (for example by saying 'oo–oo' then twisting a high pitched rattle respectively) at a point level with, and 1 m away from, each ear in turn. The baby with normal hearing will turn his head towards the sound source.

The ears of infants failing hearing screening testing should be examined for wax or evidence of middle ear infection, and re-tested after appropriate attention. Where hearing still appears unsatisfactory, the help of an ENT department or a children's hearing clinic, with access to evoked response audiometry, should be obtained.

DEAFNESS IN CHILDHOOD

During pre-school and early school years, when good hearing is so important for social, emotional, intellectual and educational development, moderate degrees of hearing loss are common.

Affected children often have no complaints but they appear inattentive, disobedient, and noisily behaved. Performance at school deteriorates, and a chain of misunderstandings can ensue which may culminate even in juvenile delinquency.

Hearing is customarily screened at about the age 2.5 years at child development assessment ('toddler') clinics, increasingly a general practice commitment. Testing entails getting the child to play with toys in order to promote some familiarity and rapport, then asking him quietly, at 1 m from each ear in turn, to perform something with the toys, for example 'put the ball in the box'. Although some idea of hearing in each ear may be gained, it is difficult to exclude unilateral problems, and results also depend on the child's co-operation and comprehension.

Thereafter routine screening, on school entry and subsequently, is a function of school medical services.

The great majority of deaf children are brought to the surgery, often for some other reason such as upper respiratory tract infections, breathing difficulties, behaviour or speech problems, or merely for routine immunisation. The general practitioner who seizes the opportunity of detecting deafness in these children, using a combination of alertness and simple examination, facilitated by a friendly rapport already established with the patient and his mother, can take steps to correct the problem long before it is belatedly discovered at a screening session.

Causes of deafness in children

Glue ear (p. 39) is much the commonest cause.

In acute otitis media (p. 28) deafness usually lasts only 1 or 2 weeks, although in a minority of cases a small amount of effusion, and some impairment of hearing, may persist for 6 weeks or more.

Wax in the meatus, even if only responsible for a 10–15 dB hearing loss, may transform a slight and acceptable hearing loss into a significant handicap. It should be removed, either by syringing after softening with Sodium Bicarbonate Ear Drops BPC or by using a wax hook or cotton wool pledget on a Jobson Horne probe. After removal of wax, regular instillation of Sodium Bicarbonate Ear Drops BPC twice/week will often prevent reaccumulation.

Mumps

This is a cause of permanent sensorineural deafness. In a survey of mumps in Islington, Fuller (1967, pers comm) encountered sensorineural deafness as a complication in 2%, predisposing to traffic accidents. A peculiarity of sensorineural deafness following mumps is that it tends to affect one ear much more than the other. The child may be unaware of his problem, hence his vulnerability to approaching traffic on his deaf side. It is a wise practice to advise parents with children suffering from mumps to check the hearing in both ears (for example using a wrist watch) 1 month after infection. If deafness is unilateral, arrangements should be made for him to sit near the front of the class, on the appropriate side, at school. He must be cautioned about the traffic danger on the deaf side. Where hearing is seriously impaired in both ears a hearing aid is essential.

Education of deaf children

Whilst special provision is initially required for seriously deaf children, the sooner they can be intergrated into a normal school system the better equipped they will be to cope with life in the community when they grow up. Ideally a teacher with special training in problems of deaf children will be appointed to ordinary schools. She will keep in regular contact with the children concerned, ensuring that their aids are satisfactory, monitoring their progress in their different classes, and devoting sessions to their special problems. Radio aids are invaluable. Since ENT clinics may be remote, the support of a local general practitioner over the care of the ears may be needed.

Every encouragement should be given to deaf children to pursue higher education if they wish. Several universities are making specific provision for deaf students, and profoundly deaf students have graduated in faculties including medicine at universities where alas no special facilities existed.

DEAFNESS IN ADULTS

Introduction

As adult life proceeds, an increasing array of threats to hearing is encountered. Many diseases may damage hearing, including the following:

Infections – particularly meningitis, septicaemia, and syphilis.

Cardiovascular diseases – especially arteriosclerosis or embolism affecting the cochlear blood supply or higher auditory pathways.

Blood disorders – including polycythemia (of rubra vera or stress type) and leukaemia.

Head injury – especially skull fracture involving the petrous temporal bone, may result in permanent deafness.

Hearing may be damaged by ototoxic drugs given systemically, particularly aminoglycoside antibiotics, ethacrynic acid, and frusemide diuretics (especially in high dose intravenously), cytotoxic drugs (especially Nitrogen mustard) and quinine. The aminoglycoside antibiotics, and others including chloramphenicol, tetracycline and erythromycin, and chlorhexidine (Hibitane) are all potentially ototoxic when placed in the middle ear. (Chloramphenicol poses the least threat, and in any case the infection for which the topical drugs are used may also be ototoxic.)

Several forms of hereditary sensorineural deafness do not become apparent until adult life.

Incidence

No precise incidence of deafness can be given, for of course there is a spectrum of hearing loss ranging from the trivial to the profound. The last survey of the prevalence of deafness in adults in Great Britain was conducted by the Central Office of Information in 1947 at the request of the Medical Research Council. The Office estimated the number of persons over 16 years of age with very severe hearing impairment (inability to hear speech at all, even with amplification) as 45 000 and of less severe deafness (down to and including difficulty in hearing in public places or in group conversation) 1 720 000. The Statistics and Research Division of the DHSS updated these figures to take account of changes in age composition of the population in 1975 and arrived at the figures shown in Table 5.2.

Table 5.2. Estimated age distribution of deaf adults.

Age (years)	Very severe impairment (thousands)	Less severe deafness (thousands)	Total (thousands)
16–44	15	333	348
45–64	19	681	700
Over 65	28	1284	1312
Total	62	2298	2360

Local authorities keep registers of both classes of hearing impairment, but figures are very incomplete as far as the lesser degrees of deafness are concerned (Table 5.3).

Table 5.3. Comparison of estimated and registered deaf per thousand population.

Class	Estimated numbers	Registered numbers (England)
Very severe impairment	1.5	0.55
Less severe impairment	55.9	0.45
Total	57.4	1.00

Otosclerosis

The term 'otosclerosis', introduced by Politzer in 1894, is misleading since the pathological process involved is a disturbance of ossification of bone embryologically derived from the otic capsule, in which mature bone is removed by osteoclasts and replaced by thick vascular unorganised bone. The resulting redness may sometimes be discernable through the t.m.: Schwartze's sign. The alternative name 'otospongiosis' is more fitting.

Whilst sporadic cases occur, this progressive disease is usually inherited as an autosomal dominant characteristic. Penetrance is very variable as is also progression of the deafness. Onset is usually in early adult life. Incidence has been put at 0.3% (Morrison, 1967). This figure relates to cases where the spongiosis process has involved the stapes footplate, fusing it to the surrounding window and causing conductive deafness. The same process may spare the stapes footplate and be confined to the cochlea, causing sensorineural deafness. In these circumstances the true cause of deafness may not be suspected. 'Stapedial' and 'cochlear' otosclerosis combined are the commonest single cause of severe adult deafness (Morrison, 1969).

Deafness in otosclerosis is usually bilateral, and often accompanied by tinnitus and sometimes by transient vertigo. Patients often speak quietly for the sound of their own voice is exaggerated by bone conduction. Paracusis occurs: conversation is heard better in noisy places. This happens because the other person raises his voice to overcome the background noise which the otosclerotic patient himself cannot hear.

The hearing loss tends to increase in one pregnancy – but strangely multiple pregnancies do not have a cumulative effect on deafness.

Detection

Because otosclerotic deafness is so amenable to relief, early recognition is important. The diagnosis should be suspected in any deaf adult with tympanic membranes of normal appearance, and tuning fork tests should be performed. Negative Rinne tests in a patient with tympanic membranes of normal appearance make the diagnosis of otosclerosis extremely likely. (But beware 'false' negative Rinne test, p. 72).

Enquiry will often reveal a family history of deafness in early adult life treated by surgery.

An audiogram serves to confirm the diagnosis; typically there is a small sensorineural loss with a larger conductive loss (Fig. 5.11). There is often a dip in hearing around 2000 Hz (Carhart's notch). The space between lines on the audiogram representing sensorineural loss above, and conductive loss below, is referred to as the air–bone gap, and this the surgeon seeks to close in the operation of stapedectomy.

Management

Surgical management. The operation of fenestration was introduced in 1914. A mastoidectomy type cavity was created with re-

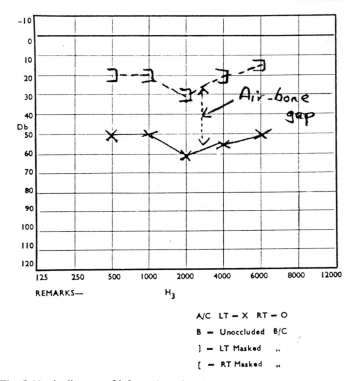

Fig. 5.11. Audiogram of left ear (otosclerosis).

moval of the ossicles, bone over the lateral semicircular canal was removed to provide a route for entry of sound into the inner ear, and a piece of the t.m. was replaced so as to create a small 'middle ear cavity' into which sound could still be 'ventilated' through the round window.

Sacrifice of the ossicles restricted the hearing improvement available from the operation, and the patient was left with a mastoid cavity with all the inconvenience this can bring.

In 1952 the introduction of the stapes mobilisation operation ended the era of fenestration surgery. This method achieved worldwide popularity, but improvement in hearing was often short-lived as the footplate became refixed.

In 1958 Shea of Memphis, Tennessee, introduced the operation of stapedectomy in which, through a transmeatal approach, the stapes was removed, the oval window covered with a vein graft, and a polythene 'stapes' was fitted between the incus and oval window to restore continuity. This operation (with various modifications such as using wire and fat, or part of the stapes itself, to restore the ossicular chain, and removing only a portion of the stapes footplate) is the basis of modern otosclerosis surgery and has enjoyed enduring success. Not only is the air bone gap usually closed, but the sensorineural loss for some unknown reason is often improved. The only serious complication of stapedectomy is perilymph fistula: leakage of perilymph through the oval window graft. This may happen immediately after operation, or at any time up to many years later. In expert hands the incidence is between 1 and 2 %. A serious leak may lead to complete loss of cochlear function: 'dead ear'. Smaller leaks give rise to fluctuation hearing loss: the middle ear should be re-opened urgently and the leak plugged. The presence of a fistula enables infection to enter the inner ear and fatal meningitis has occurred.

Medical management. In 25% of cases of otosclerosis sensorineural loss becomes stabilised spontaneously. In 75 % it progresses, and treatment with fluoride has been claimed to arrest deterioration in 80% of these (Shambaugh & Causse, 1974). Beales (1981); ENT surgeon, author of the monograph 'Otosclerosis' and leading authority on the subject in Britain, considers there is good evidence that progressive sensorineural deafness in patients who have had a successful operation and in patients who rely on a hearing aid, may be stabilised or even improved by fluoride medication. He considers fluoride safe and helpful, yet it is rarely used in this country in otosclerosis, perhaps because the subject has become emotive in connection with prevention of dental caries. A permanent maintenance dose of 20 mg of sodium fluoride daily in enteric coated form has been recommended.

Otosclerosis and the general practitioner

Diagnosis. The general practitioner, using whispering tests, otoscope, and a tuning fork (to confirm presence of hearing loss, healthy tympanic membranes, and negative Rinne test) can diagnose otosclerosis with moderate confidence. With a characteristic audiogram and a family history of otosclerosis little doubt remains.

Referral. Results of surgery are so good that operation should be advised in patients diagnosed at almost any age. In the 1960s a large number of unoperated cases existed and as these came to surgery many ENT specialists became experienced and competent in stapes surgery. Techniques have advanced in this difficult and specialised branch of ENT surgery, and since there is now but a trickle of new patients coming forward for stapedectomy, it is best that general practitioners refer them to major ENT centres where sufficient practice is available for skills to be maintained.

Counselling. Stay in hospital for stapedectomy is less than 1 week. Post-operatively, giddiness is usual for a few days. After stapedectomy patients can be encouraged to swim, but not to dive, lift heavy objects, or blow their noses violently. Trips to mountains and flying unfortunately increase the risk of perilymph fistula, and many patients elect to forgo these. Any patient complaining of sudden hearing deterioration should be referred back to the ENT surgeon immediately, as a perilymph fistula is likely.

Patients delighted with the results of surgery on one ear may be anxious to have the other ear operated upon. In general this is discouraged – the risk of late perilymph fistula always exists and it is probably best to preserve one ear to benefit from future technological advances or for a hearing aid.

Patients who have undergone fenestration operations

Most are now old age pensioners. Their cavities should be examined once or twice a year and cleaned if necessary, either by an interested general practitioner or in the hospital out-patient department. Most will require a hearing aid. It is occasionally possible to improve hearing with a modified form of 'stapedectomy' after fenestration.

Otosclerosis and the 'pill'

In view of the adverse effect of pregnancy in otosclerosis, the advisability of oral contraception has been questioned. Pharmaceutical literature accompanying combined oral contraceptive preparations quotes hearing loss from otosclerosis as a contra-indication, and MIMS gives 'deterioration of otosclerosis during pregnancy' as a contra-indication to combined oral contraceptives but not to progesterone-only contraceptives.

MENIÈRE'S DISEASE

In 1861 Prosper Menière described a disease consisting of the triad of sudden and recurring attacks of vertigo (often accompanied by nausea and vomiting), tinnitus, and fluctuating deafness. He suspected the cause lay in the labyrinth. In 1938 Hallpike and Cairns published post mortem findings confirming this with gross distension and rupture of the scala media (Fig. 5.12). The reason for this distension (endolymphatic hydrops) remains unknown. It is uncertain whether excessive production or diminished absorption, or both, are responsible. Nor is it certain whether attacks are initiated or relieved when the distended scale media finally ruptures, and endolymph and perilymph become intermixed. An association has been noted between Menière's triad of symptoms and certain conditions which have consequently been postulated to be aetiological. These include syphilis, migraine, head injury, otosclerosis, allergy, hypothyroidism, narrow internal auditory meatus, glucose intolerance, viral infections, and Paget's disease. In one study of 120 cases (Pulec, 1977) a specific aetiology was considered identifiable in 55%, and the remaining 45% were idiopathic. Idiopathic cases are often said to be suffering from Menière's *disease*, whilst the term Menière's *syndrome* is used for patients in whom a presumptive cause is identified.

Males are affected more often than females, and most first attacks occur before the age of 50 years.

The *incidence* of Menière's disease is unknown. 0.5 per cent of patients attending ENT clinics for any reason suffered from the disease in one study involving hospitals in several countries (Matsunaga, 1976). A survey in Sweden indicated the disease to be four times as common as otosclerosis (Stahle et al, 1978). Over one-half of all cases of vertigo referred to ENT departments prove to have Menière's disease. However many patients are seen in general practice with attacks of giddiness so easily controlled and so infrequent that further investigations are not undertaken.

Incidence of bilateral involvement

The disease usually affects one ear only for many years but eventually both sides may become involved. In one specialist centre 42.5 % of cases had become bilateral after 20 years (Morrison, 1975).

Clinical course

Many patients have a small number of attacks, after which the disease appears to be arrested with no sequelae other than a variable

DEAFNESS 93

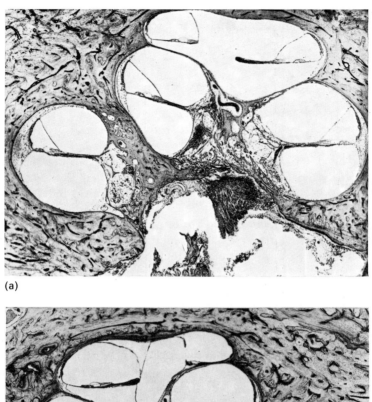

(a)

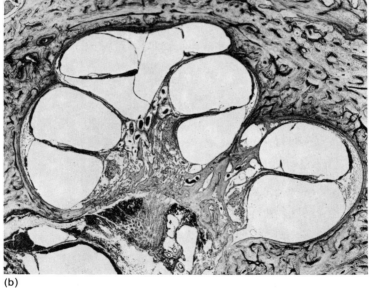

(b)

Fig. 5.12.(a) Normal cochlea (the unaffected side of a case of Menière's disease); (b) left cochlea affected by Menière's disease showing gross dilatation of the scala media with displacement of Reissner's membrane through the helicotrema. (Reproduced by courtesy of the Royal Society of Medicine and Mr Bernard Colman).

degree of deafness. At the other end of the spectrum frequent severe attacks occur, resulting in prolonged incapacitation and serious hearing loss.

Clinical picture

The patient during an attack of Menière's disease is likely to be in considerable distress, lying still, with a basin near at hand for vomiting into. Nystagmus is usually present.

Examination of the ear, apart perhaps from revealing sensori-neural deafness, is negative, as is also examination of the central nervous system. (Serious pathology such as posterior inferior cerebellar artery thrombosis must be excluded).

The attacks of giddiness tend to be accompanied by tinnitus and deafness which at first ease after 1 or 2 days, but later become more persistent. Severe cases become profoundly deaf and the tinnitus may become very distressing, often likened to a dynamo.

Associated with attacks, the patient may also complain of distortion of hearing and an uncomfortable 'full' feeling in the ear. The distended saccule may press against the oval window with the result that loud sounds produce giddiness: the Tullio phenomenon. If this is not understood some of the patient's symptoms may be dismissed as functional.

Diagnosis

The history given by a patient with Menière's disease is often so characteristic as to be diagnostic. However one or more components of the triad of giddiness, tinnitus, and deafness may be absent, especially initially but sometimes throughout. An audiogram should be performed, partly for diagnosis (a principally low-tone sensorineural loss is characteristic) and partly as a 'base-line' for future comparison.

Where diagnosis is uncertain, and especially if surgical treatment is contemplated, hospital investigations will include sophisticated audiometry, caloric tests of vestibular function, X-ray tomography and electrocochleography and/or brain-stem electric response audiometry. The effects of profound dehydration with glycerol are studied in some centres: endolymph pressure is reduced, and improvement in pure tone audiometry supports the diagnosis.

Differential diagnosis

The clinical picture in sudden vestibular failure (p. 127) may closely resemble an attack of Menière's disease: a firm diagnosis may only be possible in retrospect.

Initially posterior inferior cerebellar artery thrombosis may give a clinical picture resembling an acute attack of Menière's disease but further neurological complications supervene.

Conditions mentioned as causes of Menière's syndrome should be excluded.

Medical management

Patients suffering from Menière's disease are liable to become extremely worried and distressed. They are rendered helpless during attacks, and become fearful of further episodes. Anxiety sometimes appears instrumental in triggering further attacks. They may need strong reassurance that they have a non-fatal self limiting condition which can be helped by medical treatment and for which surgical help is available in the very small minority of cases who eventually need it.

During the *acute attack* intramuscular prochlorperazine (Stemetil) 12.5 mg, or chlorpromazine (Largactil) 50–100 mg should be administered and repeated as necessary. Attacks may be lessened in frequency and severity, if not prevented, by betahistine (Serc), one or two 8 mg tablets daily as long-term maintenance therapy (the drug is claimed to lower endolymph pressure). Prochlorperazine (Stemetil) 5 mg three times/day and cinnarizine (Stugeron) 15 mg three times/day are also widely used.

Dietary restrictions and vasodilator drugs have been generally abandoned as useless.

Surgical management

Where medical measures fail various surgical procedures are available. For reasons not understood, the mere insertion of a grommet into the t.m. appears to reduce attacks in some patients and should always be tried.

For patients with disabling attacks of vertigo who have already lost all useful hearing in the ear, simple destruction of the entire labyrinth has long been practised.

Where useful hearing remains, division of the vestibular portion of the 8th nerve at the base of the brain has been advocated. The operation is hazardous and does nothing to alter the progression of the disease.

Modern surgery is designed to provide endolymph drainage so that damaging distension of the labyrinth is prevented and the disease arrested. For many years attention has focused on the saccus endolymphaticus (p. 63). Patients with Menière's disease have narrowed or obliterated sacs. Mere exposure of the saccus end, by removal of surrounding bone, has its advocates. Others advise insertion of a unidirectional microvalve (originally developed for glaucoma) allowing endolymph to drain into the mastoid space.

Few ENT surgeons are now convinced that saccus surgery has anything but a placebo effect. In a study in Denmark 30 patients with Menière's disease were divided into two groups (Thomsen et al, 1981). Half received saccus drainage operations whilst the other half had mastoid operations but the saccus was not approached. Neither the patients nor the observers knew which had had 'proper' and which 'placebo' operations. Careful follow-up at the end of 1 year revealed little difference between the progress of either group. Both groups in fact improved significantly. (This study, incidentally, was initiated before the Helsinki declaration on medical ethics became effective in Denmark. Such studies would presumably no longer be permissible.)

More recently the operation of cochleostomy has been advocated. Since this operation involves creating an artificial fistula between endolymph and perilymph, its physiological soundness appears questionable.

Menière's disease and the general practitioner

Patients with Menière's disease present a dilemma. The great majority will be helped by medication and reassurance. A very small minority will continue with disabling attacks of vertigo and deteriorating hearing. Only the passage of time can identify this group. For them saccus surgery, albeit probably merely a placebo, may offer the best hope of relief and the general practitioner should refer them to a centre where this is available.

Patients with unilateral deafness should also be referred, particulary to exclude the presence of an acoustic neuroma.

NOISE-INDUCED HEARING LOSS

Effects of excessive noise on the ear

The cochlea is vulnerable to noise and may be damaged by a very loud sound of short duration or a less intense sound over a longer period.

A temporary threshold shift occurs where exposure to loud sounds results in temporary hearing loss. Whatever the frequency of the stimulus, the hearing loss begins to appear at about 4000 Hz and spreads to involve frequencies above and below, producing a 'notch' in an audiogram deepest at 4000 Hz. The depth and duration of a temporary threshold shift varies with the intensity and duration of the stimulus, but higher stimulus frequencies tend to have more effect than lower frequencies of the same loudness and duration.

In general a 2-hour exposure to a 70–75 dB sound at 1000 Hz is required to produce a temporary threshold shift. Exposure to a 1000 Hz sound at 120 dB for 30 min is commonly followed by a temporary threshold shift of 35 dB which recovers the following day.

Individuals show marked variation in tolerance to noise. Temporary threshold shifts tend to return to normal after 1 or 2 days. Any improvement after 2 days is likely to be small and very slow (a different situation is encountered in massive threshold shifts resulting from explosion, where recovery may continue for several weeks).

During recovery, the notch recorded in serial audiograms becomes progressively shallower. The dip at 4000 Hz is the last to recover.

Permanent threshold shift

Temporary threshold shifts may merge into permanent shifts, but the relationship is inconstant and individually variable. For the same noise exposure one person may respond with a temporary threshold shift whilst another may never fully recover: some of the shift is permanent (Fig. 5.13)

This individual variability greatly complicates the subject of noise induced deafness. In industry, sport, the armed services, and music, agreement has proved virtually impossible to reach on a level of noise exposure 'safe' for any individual. It is widely accepted that

98 EAR, NOSE AND THROAT DISORDERS

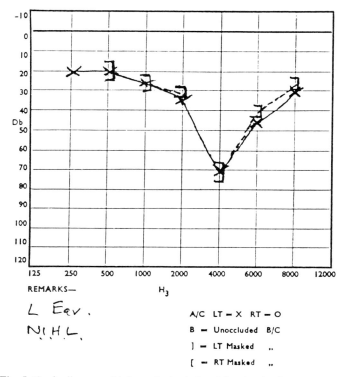

Fig. 5.13. Audiogram of left ear (noise induced hearing loss).

exposures to noise of 90 dBA (the 'A' refers to the filter used on the sound level meter) during a working week of 40 hours is 'safe'. However this is only true for 85 % of the population, and 15 % of people exposed to this sound level over a prolonged period will develop permanent deafness. To protect 95 % of exposed persons, an 85 dBA 'safe' level must be used. (These figures assume that no hearing protectors are worn.) To achieve this degree of sound-proofing in many industrial settings is extremely difficult and expensive. Even then, 5 % of workers remain at risk.

Whilst a few industrial processes involve steady noise intensity, in most, noise is intermittent, irregular, and difficult or impossible to meter satisfactorily. Brief, harmful percussion-like sounds may be too short lived to register on even the most modern sound meter. There is plainly a wide area for potential disputes between employers and unions.

Sources of excessive noise

Printing, drop forging, textile manufacture, glass bottle handling processes, mining, electricity generation and tractor driving are amongst occupations carrying special risks to hearing.

The danger to hearing of loud noise has been known for centuries, yet despite codes of practice, legislation governing safety, preventative measures, and compensation legislation, noise induced hearing loss continues. People in noisy occupations tend to be well paid, and may tolerate harmfully loud noise too readily. They often neglect to wear ear protectors, on the grounds that prolonged wearing of these is too uncomfortable and impracticable.

Ear damage from explosions

Most victims of blast injury have sensorineural deafness, together with tinnitus, but many recover, either rapidly or over the course of a few weeks.

Small arms fire is a potent cause of permanent hearing loss; in the case of rifle shooting the forward ear is chiefly affected, the ear away from the muzzle being protected in the 'head shadow'. Pistol shooting characteristically damages both ears equally.

Deafness from music

Discotheques and pop concerts, with their powerful amplification, are obvious danger areas. The risks have extensively studied with the general conclusion that occasional attendance is unlikely to cause significant lasting damage to hearing, but that professional musicians and regular devotees are liable to suffer permanent hearing loss. Symphony orchestra players have also been shown to risk noise induced hearing loss. In one study (Westmere & Fuersden, 1981) involving principal orchestras in London, noise-induced hearing loss was present in just over one-third of the ears tested (representatives from all orchestral sections were examined). Members of the woodwind section (usually seated in front of the brass and percussion sections) were most severely affected. Many musicians protect their ears with plugs. Clarinetists have particular problems since their cochleae have a direct physical contact with the sound source via the mouthpiece and upper teeth. They are unable to use earplugs as this restricts their hearing to mere buzzing from the reed, preventing them monitoring the air conducted sounds they are making.

Presentation of noise induced hearing loss

Noise induced hearing loss can be detected by screening long before symptoms develop. The 4000 Hz dip may be present and gradually extending for years, as the patient continues his exposure to loud noise quite oblivious that anything is wrong. Eventually the 'lower' side of the dip spreads to involve the speech frequencies (1000–2000 Hz) and awareness of a handicap may begin. The first complaint is often of difficulty in following conversations, especially in the presence of background noise. Deafness gradually increases and when, with the passage of years, presbycusis is super-added the patient may be severely handicapped.

Role of the general practitioner

Employers in industries liable to cause noise induced hearing loss are increasingly taking steps to monitor those at risk, reduce sound emission, and provide and encourage the use of ear protectors.

The workers themselves are not always fully appreciative of the risks they run, and anything the general practitioner can do to emphasise the importance of co-operation with these measures is helpful. For many workers at risk there is little or no provision for screening or prevention, and of course in many cases the injury to hearing occurs during leisure or sporting pursuits.

The general practitioner with an audiometer can render a valuable service to those of his patients likely to be at risk of noise induced hearing loss through occupational or other loud noise. A periodic audiogram, annually or less frequently depending on the degree of risk, will pick up the characteristic 4000 Hz 'dip' long before the patient is aware anything is wrong, and in good time to take avoiding action before serious deafness has developed.

Entitlement to disablement benefit for occupational deafness

The general practitioner's advice may be sought (or volunteered) regarding the likelihood of success in an application for disablement benefit. The requirements are rigorous. The worker must have been employed in a 'prescribed' occupation for 20 years, and broadly he may hope to obtain a disability payment ranging from 20 %, if his hearing loss attributed to the occupation is 50 dB, up to 100 % if the attributed loss is 110 dB.

If he appears eligible for industrial compensation, the patient should be encouraged to approach the local office of the DHSS without delay, since a further requirement is that the worker must have been employed in the 'prescribed' occupation within 1 year of the claim being made. The Industrial Injuries Advisory Council has had under consideration relaxation of these requirements, possibly with a reduction of the minimum working period from 20 to 10 years, and extension of the list of 'prescribed' occupations. New regulations appear imminent, so workers with 10 years' exposure should also be encouraged to submit a claim to the DHSS. The DHSS make enquiries to confirm that the occupational requirements are met, arrange for an otologist's report, then convene a medical board to decide the validity of the claim and to assess 'percentage disablement' guided by tables agreed with the British Association of Otolaryngologists.

SUDDEN SENSORINEURAL HEARING LOSS

Introduction

The sudden development of sensorineural deafness should be looked upon as an ENT emergency.

It is a relatively rare event. The true incidence is not ascertainable since medical advice is often not sought at the time, particularly where the loss is unilateral. Individual general practitioners are unlikely to see more than a handful of cases in a working life. An understandable consequence of lack of familiarity with the condition is that it is not always handled with appropriate urgency.

Aetiology

The site of the lesion responsible for sudden sensorineural loss may be in the cochlea, 8th nerve, or brain. In only a minority of cases is the cause apparent.

Cochlear causes

These include the following:
1. *Infections – viral and bacterial.* Mumps is the commonest viral agent (see page 85) and since the hearing loss is usually severe on

one side only, it may go unnoticed until uncovered by a road accident, at a medical examination prompted by poor school performance, or merely at routine screening. The mumps antibody titre should always be measured in cases of unexplained sudden hearing loss.

Measles and herpes zoster virus are also causes of sudden sensorineural hearing loss.

Bacterial infection may destroy the cochlea as a result of extension of chronic suppurative otitis media, principally in the presence of cholesteatoma.

Syphilis, congenital or acquired, may invade the cochlea causing sudden deafness. The hearing loss is typically asymmetrical, but often severe on both sides. Diagnosis is by history, clinical examination for stigmata, and by serology. Unfortunately in late syphilis the routine screening tests, including the cardiolipin Wassermann reaction (CWR), VDRL test, and Reiter protein complement fixation tests are often negative. The fluorescent treponemal antibody test is the most sensitive. Treatment is by combined penicillin and prednisone. A protocol involving hospital admission for a 17-day course of intramuscular penicillin G 500 000 units 6-hourly, combined with prednisone 10 mg three times/day by mouth for one week then 25 mg/day for 3 weeks has been recommended (Morrison, 1975).

2. *Trauma.* The cochlea may be damaged as a result of fracture of the base of the skull involving the temporal bone. During the first few weeks some recovery may occur. Sensorineural loss may occur in patients struck by lightning.

3. *Perilymph leak* from a rupture of round or oval windows is an increasingly recognised cause of sudden sensorineural hearing loss. Such rupture is seen in underwater divers, but may occur as a result of a minor incident such as coughing or sneezing. The resulting fall in perilymph pressure may damage the cochlea, and also permits entry of infection into the inner ear with resulting labyrinthitis. Where the sequence of events suggests perilymph leak, urgent admission to a fully equipped ENT unit is essential so that the hearing loss can be investigated and monitored, and any leak identified and arrested by plugging.

4. *Radiotherapy* to head and neck neoplasms may lead to cochlear damage and sensorineural deafness sometimes only manifest many years later.

5. *Menière's Disease.* This may rarely present with sudden sensorineural deafness.

6. *Vascular causes of sudden sensorineural hearing loss.* The cochlear vessels are derived from the internal auditory artery. This vessel receives blood from the vertebral artery by a variable route. In 10 % of cases, all the blood to both inner ears is derived from one vertebral artery, the other terminating in the neck. The effects on hearing of vascular spasm, haemorrhage, or occlusion from embolism may therefore vary greatly, and are sometimes catastrophic. The ear may be affected by all the underlying conditions leading to cerebrovascular accidents.

7. *Haematological causes* include polycythemia of the vera or 'stress' types. Increased viscosity leads to sludging and cochlear anoxia. The leukaemias, macroglobulinaemias and haemoglobinopathies may also cause vascular plugging.

8. *Drug induced deafness.* Ototoxicity, especially from aminoglycoside antibiotics (particularly kanamycin, neomycin, tobramycin and dihydrostreptomycin) may give rise to sudden hearing loss. Streptomycin and gentamycin may also cause cochlear damage but affect the vestibular apparatus more often.

9. *Ethnacrynic acid.* This may cause cochlear damage when given intravenously or in the presence of renal failure. The loss is sometimes reversible. Administration of frusemide carries similar risks.

Retrocochlear causes

Meningitis (pyogenic, tubercular, or viral) may damage the 8th nerve leading to sudden hearing loss. Tumour involvement, including acoustic neuroma and secondary carcinoma, may also be responsible.

Idiopathic sudden sensorineural deafness

Most cases fall into this category. Onset is often accompanied by discomfort in the ear, tinnitus, and vertigo. The cause is presumed to be either viral or vascular.

In view of the uncertainty as to cause, management remains controversial. Some believe most cases are of vascular origin, and advocate administration of vasodilators, intravenous histamine drip, and stellate ganglion block.

Those who favour a viral aetiology recommend immediate administration of steroids, and most authorities consider this the correct management in idiopathic cases where the lesion appears most likely to be retrocochlear. In one series, 90 % of cases improved when treatment was initiated during the first week, whereas none improved if treatment was delayed for 1 month or more (Morrison, 1975).

Management in general practice

The general practitioner encountering a patient with sudden onset of sensorineural deafness should arrange his immediate referral to a well equipped ENT for full investigation. A treatable cause may be identifiable, leading to salvage of hearing. Where no cause is ascertainable, and particularly where investigations suggest a retrocochlear lesion, administration of steroids (such as Prednisone on a reducing dosage starting at 60 mg/day) is currently the treatment of choice.

If delay in transfer to a specialist unit is unavoidable, the general practitioner might be well advised to initiate steroid therapy as a 'first aid' procedure. As Morrison (1975) points out, even if the patient is later found to have an acoustic neuroma, late syphilis, or endolymphatic hydrops, or even psychogenic deafness, treatment can be withdrawn 'whereas a few days' delay may affect the ultimate results in sensorineural deafness. This is one of the occasions when slavery to diagnosis must be avoided'.

PRESBYCUSIS

Introduction

The term presbycusis refers to the hearing loss consequent upon aging processes (Fig. 5.14). These chiefly affect the cochlea, but may also be significant in the central auditory pathway. The deafness is characteristically bilaterally symmetrical, and affects high tones predominantly.

By this time of life the ear may already have been affected by one or more other causes of hearing loss. Supervening presbycusis is frequently only partially responsible for an elderly person's hearing difficulty. The time of onset and rate of progress of the ageing processes responsible for presbycusis appear to be governed to some extent by the sum of background noise experienced over the years. Presbycusis appears to begin earlier in urban than in rural communities (Rosen et al, 1964). Philipzoon (1962) reported the case of an elderly man who had deliberately worn a cotton wool plug in one ear for 32 years. The audiogram for high tones in this ear was much better than in the unprotected ear.

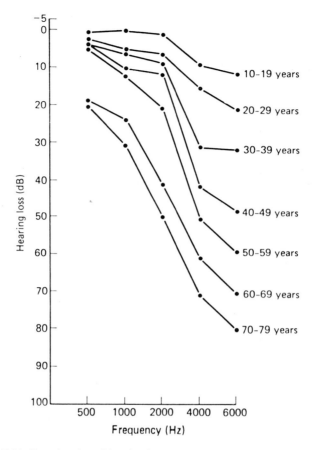

Fig. 5.14. Deterioration of hearing in progressive decades.

Hearing loss predominant for high tones has been explained on the grounds that they are appreciated in the basal turn of the cochlea, whilst lower turns are appreciated higher up in the cochlear spiral. Being nearest the oval window, through which vibrations enter the cochlea, the basal turn bears the brunt of 'wear and tear' and hearing for high tones fails first.

Pathology

Changes have been demonstrated predominantly affecting any of four different sites in the cochlea (Fig. 5.15).

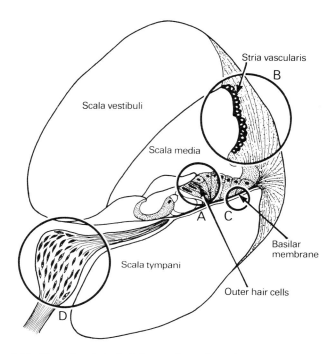

Fig. 5.15. Sites of pathological changes in preshycusis.

a. In 'sensory presbycusis' there is atrophy of the organ of Corti in the basal turn of the cochlea, with disappearance of hair cells.

b. In 'strial presbycusis' there is patchy atrophy of the stria vascularis, with cystic changes.

c. In 'cochlear conductive presbycusis' the basilar membrane becomes stiffened and calcified, especially in the basal turn.

d. In 'neural presbycusis' there is atrophy of the spiral ganglion with severe loss of ganglion cells.

Audiograms have been correlated with subsequent post-mortem studies, and reveal that neural presbycusis is associated with severe loss of speech discrimination, and strial presbycusis with audiograms showing a fairly even hearing loss at all frequencies with good speech discrimination. High tone loss is characteristic of the sensory and cochlear conductive forms.

Atrophic changes in the central auditory pathway are also present in many elderly patients suffering from hearing difficulties.

Clinical features

The characteristic slowly progressive bilateral high tone hearing loss is often accompanied by continuous high pitched tinnitus. This often leads the patient to seek medical advice (perhaps fearing he has high blood pressure or even a tumour) long before he is aware of any hearing loss. Patients commonly exhibit the phenomenon of recruitment (p. 70) and this may add to problems with hearing aid wearing.

Diagnosis

The t.m. is usually of normal appearance in presbycusis, and examination with a tuning fork reveals a positive Rinne test on both sides with no lateralisation in the Weber test.

Pure tone audiometry usually clinches the diagnosis, revealing a symmetrical high tone loss which gradually extends to involve lower frequencies with the passage of years. It is only when speech frequencies (1000-2000 Hz) become involved that there is much conversational difficulty.

In 1957 a wide survey of hearing at different decades in Winsconsin State, USA, established standard curves for hearing loss due to age (Fig. 5.14).

Management

Accumulation of wax often increases the degree of handicap in presbycusis, and periodic removal of this may help the patient considerably. When hearing loss at speech frequencies approaches 40 dB, a hearing aid trial should be arranged. Patients with deeply sloping audiograms sometimes find electric aids unhelpful – it is difficult even with modern selective aids to achieve satisfactory amplification of high tones without excessive amplification of lower tones, leading to distortion. Where presbycusis involves predominantly the spiral ganglion or central auditory pathway, a hearing aid may merely serve to amplify distorted hearing, explaining the patients unwillingness to use it. An old fashioned speaking tube, providing a 20dB gain, sometimes gives the best results.

CONSEQUENCES OF DEAFNESS

Loss of hearing is a particularly distressing handicap. Not only is life impoverished when music, the singing of birds, and the greetings of friends cannot be heard, but, even worse, the impairment of communication is likely to lead to an increasing feeling of isolation, withdrawal, and depression.

Unlike the handicap of blindness, which attracts instant sympathy, benevolence, and a desire to help from all around, deafness tends to provoke irritation, impatience and exasperation. Blind people are, in general, serene and happy compared with the deaf who are all too often misunderstood, lonely, and miserable.

Furthermore, provision of community support for the deaf lags well behind that for the blind. A sub-committee of the DHSS Advisory Committee on Services for Hearing Impaired People (ACSHIP), set up in 1974 to consider the rehabilitation of the adult hearing impaired, commented: 'It is barely credible that, in the affluent society in which we have lived during the past 25 years so little has been done'.

Problems within the family

Hearing difficulties in the home environment frequently lead to consultations in general practice. This may vary from good-natured banter 'He says he's deaf, but he can hear perfectly well when he wants to',through stages of more serious misunderstanding and disagreement, 'He wants the television on so loud I can't stand it, and he never listens to me when I speak to him', to a state of severe breakdown of inter-personal relationships. The deaf person sometimes becomes quite paranoid, wrongly believing that people are talking disparagingly about him, and jeering at him, and that he is no longer wanted in the home. Much of what deaf people say when attempting to join a conversation is likely to be inappropriate and may appear laughable. The sufferer may soon feel he is the subject of ridicule. As deafness largely precludes normal social and recreational activities, distress when the atmosphere at home degenerates can be profound. Tinnitus is a common accompaniment to deafness, compounding the patient's misery. Without understanding, patience, and goodwill from those around him, a previously pleasant personality may degenerate to leave the deaf person isolated, bitter and hostile.

Where the patient lives alone there are of course additional problems, and the sense of isolation may be extreme. Deafness represents a safety risk, particularly from road accidents.

The general practitioner can usually do much to help. Simple discussion with exasperated relatives will often improve their understanding of the deaf patient's problems and help to defuse matters. An induction loop for a television socket, enabling the patient to hear programmes with the set either silent or adjusted to normal volume, to suit relatives with normal hearing, can be of immense help (see page 118). The patient's hearing aid should be checked, and the external meatus inspected for wax or debris. Relatives should be reminded that the patient is likely to be relying largely on lip reading, so that they should make sure their lips are visible when attempting conversation. Speech should be clear and not too fast. It is often helpful to discuss recruitment with them (page 70) in simple terms. They may then come to understand better the hitherto annoying habit of the deaf person of taking no notice of an approaching noise, such as a car, until it is almost upon them, then appearing to jump out of their skins, and of retorting ungraciously when someone raises their voice to try to get through to them, 'Don't shout at me — I'm not deaf!' Appreciation of the fact that many deaf people live in a world where they are frequently being startled by loud noises may bring a more sympathetic understanding of their plight.

Problems at work

Problems encountered by deaf people at work are unfortunately likely to increase with the passage of years and inevitable onset of high tone hearing loss. Every effort must be made to ensure that the patient's limited hearing is being exploited to the full. Periodic visits should be made to a hearing aid clinic where it may be possible to substitute better instruments as either the patient's hearing threshold rises or technological advances reach the market.

Great strides have been made in recent years in the perfection of ear level aids which can now replace the more cumbersome and inconvenient body worn aids except in the more severely handicapped. In some occupations, particularly those involving committee or conference work, it may be best to wear two aids, one in each ear.

Difficulties can arise where a person is aware of his deteriorating hearing, but is reluctant to acknowledge this or take steps to consult a doctor for reasons of vanity or a fear that the wearing of an aid might prejudice promotion prospects.

Deaf employees working in very noisy environments present a particular dilemma. The noise may be contributory, or may even be the primary cause of the deafness. Such occupations tend to be well paid, and, not being qualified for any other, the employee may be most reluctant to consider a change of job. Many workers in noisy occupations are also resistant to the idea of wearing ear protectors, considering them too uncomfortable. Whilst this is strongly to be deprecated, every effort should be made by the employer to quieten and sound-insulate noisy equipment in accordance with the code of practice introduced in 1972 and likely to form the basis of legislation through the Health and Safety Executive in the future. This code of practice proposed an exposure to 90 dBA over 8 hours as the maximum consistent with safety to the ears. Many would regard this as excessive, and TUC policy is that exposure to 70 dBA should be the maximum where concentration is required.

MANAGEMENT OF DEAFNESS

In September 1975 the sub-committee of DHSS ACSHIP set up to consider rehabilitation of the adult hearing impaired, reported their recommendations. These included the introduction of the new category of worker to be called a 'hearing therapist'. A 36-week training syllabus was proposed. The DHSS provisionally undertook to finance training for 10 hearing therapists annually in London (at the 'City Lit') starting in 1978. So far, some 50 hearing therapists have been trained, and are scattered throughout the UK attached to ENT departments. From their job description (see below) it is evident that, once their numbers are sufficient, they will rectify many of the present deficiencies in the care of deaf people. Close ties with general practitioners will be essential.

Job specification of a staff grade within the NHS to be designated 'hearing therapist'

1. A knowledge of the cause and effect of the various types and degrees of hearing impairment as a prerequisite for the overall assessment of the patient.

2. An ability to recognise the patient's need for further help in medical, technical, social, financial, environmental, vocational and educational areas as part of the rehabilitative process, and sufficient knowledge to enable the guidance of treatment as necessary.

3. An awareness of the social implications of hearing impairment; the ability to assess the degree of a patient's social handicap in relation to his hearing loss; knowledge of the measures required

to alleviate that condition and an ability to execute those measures.

4. A capability to recognise the needs of those patients requiring help beyond the level of basic instruction; assessment of the need and the provision of instruction in auditory clues, lip reading, auditory training and guidance on speech preservation in either the individual or group situation.

5. A knowledge of the range of performance of all hearing aids available under the NHS and of the effects of varying acoustic conditions, in order to ensure that the patient is able to make the most effective use of his hearing aid, in either a group or one-to-one situation.

6. A working knowledge of the simpler mechanical aspects of all hearing aids available under the NHS, recognition of the more common faults, and an ability to remedy those faults.

7. A knowledge of the range and functions of available environmental aids and equipment together with their relevance to the individual patient's needs and an ability to demonstrate a range of such aids.

8. Recognition of the need for co-operation with other statutory and voluntary agencies and the benefits and services they provide. Where appropriate, and in conjunction with the social worker, achievement of effective co-ordination with those agencies in order to secure optimum advantages and benefits for the patient's social rehabilitation.

9. A knowledge of the causes and effects of deafness at work: and an ability to liaise with employers to ensure that optimum opportunities can be secured for present and prospective employees.

10. An outline knowledge of the legislation affecting directly and indirectly the rights of patients suffering from hearing impairment.

11. A capability to introduce, maintain, direct and control an information system designed to: a. record referrals of patients requiring rehabilitation; b. record their progress; c. identify those who do not respond to appointments, with a view to ensuring appropriate follow-up action is taken in either the hospital or domiciliary situation.

Hearing therapists taking up post are overwhelmed by the workload confronting them, and in my own practice the potentialities of co-operation with attached district nurses are being examined.

Hearing aids

Any patient with a hearing loss at speech frequencies

(1000–2000 Hz) of 40 dB or more is likely to benefit from provision of a hearing aid. The general practitioner advising such a patient will normally refer him to a hospital ENT department designated for the purpose. Aids, and their accessories, are supplied to such hospitals directly by the DHSS, and their cost is thus independent of the district health budget.

Some patients with hearing difficulties consult a private hearing aid dispenser, often in response to an advertisement. A controlling body, the Hearing Aid Council, was set up by Act of Parliament to maintain a register of dispensers and to govern some of their professional activities. Regulations require that if a hearing aid dispenser discovers that a patient might have conductive deafness or features other than those of a slowly progressive bilateral sensorineural loss, he must refer the patient to his general practitioner.

The Hearing Aid Council has no control over advertising by hearing aid dispensers, and concern has been occasioned over unwarranted advertising claims. The Hearing Aid Industry Association, a voluntary body, has its own advertising committee which screens advertisements from dispensing companies to ensure that copy does not contravene the association's own rules. Despite this, in the words of the Director of the Royal National Institute for the Deaf (RNID) in 1981 'many thousands of handicapped people had their hopes dashed after buying aids which have been promoted in ways which, by any standards, are unethical'.

For many years the NHS would only provide 'Medresco' bodyworn aids for all but a small group of deaf patients. Many patients resorted to private sources to obtain much preferred post-aural aids. The NHS would not undertake repair of privately acquired aids, nor supply batteries for them. In January 1983 this policy was rationalised, and these services are now possible if endorsed by a NHS Consultant. In 1977 the NHS began to supply post-aural aids for all patients. At first the range was restricted, and deafer patients requiring more powerful post-aural aids were still obliged to purchase these privately. In 1980 high power post-aural aids became available, followed in 1981 by very high power body worn aids with facilities for air and bone conduction and further very high power post-aural models.

In obtaining an aid through the NHS the patient is saved the initial cost of the instrument (£100–£500) and the cost of batteries and repairs, and receives a proper medical ear examination. Nevertheless private dispensers sometimes, with ingenuity and flexibility, overcome special problems unresolvable through NHS channels.

Types of hearing aids

All modern hearing aids comprise a microphone, an amplifier, a gain control, and an earphone. A battery is required to power the amplifier, and nowadays an induction pick-up coil is a standard provision. A switch enables either the microphone (M position) or the induction coil (T position) to be connected to the amplifier. In addition to an on – off switch a tone control is also provided to modify amplification. The letters H, N, and L are used, denoting high frequency emphasis (low frequency cut), normal (the widest) frequency response that the aid can produce), and low frequency emphasis (high frequency cut).

Body-worn aids

These consist of a box, worn either slung from the neck or hitched to a suitable piece of clothing, containing a microphone, amplifier, pick-up coil and battery. A long lead runs from the box up to an earphone attached to an insert in the ear [Fig. 5.16(a)].

Body-worn aids are cumbersome, and the leads require fairly frequent replacement since they are liable to fracture. They are however capable of more powerful amplification than ear level aids and so are indispensible for the very deaf. Powerful body-worn aids are capable of gains of over 70 dB at 1000 Hz, with a maximum acoustic output in excess of 135 dB sound pressure level. (With the newest body-worn aids, the BW80 series, the gain can reach about 90 dB.) The corresponding figures for ear-level aids are over 60 dB and over 125 dB SPL at 1000 Hz respectively.

Ear-level aids

Three types are available.

1. Post-aural aids. these contain all the components in a curved container. A short plastic tube connects the earphone at the top of the aid to the insert in the meatus. This is much the most widely used type today. [Fig. 5.16(b)].

2. Spectacle aids. Some patients experience discomfort in wearing spectacles and a post-aural aid at the same time, and prefer a combination spectacle aid in which the parts of the aid are incorporated in the arms of the spectacles. An obvious disadvantage of this arrangement is that an accident to the instrument leaves the patient doubly handicapped.

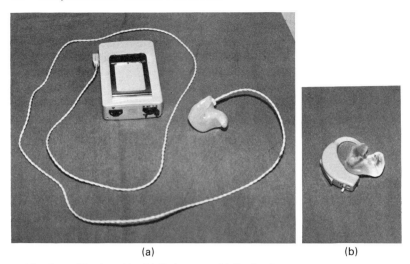

Fig. 5.16. Hearing aids. (a) Body-worn. (b) Ear-level.

3. In-the-ear aids. Increasing miniaturisation has made it possible to incorporate all the components of an aid in a unit small enough to rest in the concha of the ear, where it is attached to a conventional type of insert. This obviates any interference with spectacle arms. Some wearers feel an in-the-ear-aid to be more cosmetically acceptable, but for most a post-aural aid is less conspicuous and more satisfactory. Spectacle and in-the-ear aids are not available through the NHS.

Hearing aid microphones

These are of three main types.

1. Electromagnetic
2. Crystal or ceramic
3. Electret

All can be miniaturised sufficiently for post-aural aids. The electromagnetic type shows limited response to low frequencies. The crystal or ceramic type gives a good low frequency response but requires its own power supply to operate a field effect transistor. The electret microphone gives the best range frequency response, and greatest freedom from interference due to vibration. It uses a form of capacitor, the potential being supplied by electret material which holds a charge. The microphone is thus of limited life, although this is measured in years.

Hearing aid amplifiers

A basic problem with hearing aids is that if amplification is sufficient to render low volume sounds audible, then louder sounds may be amplified to a degree where loudness discomfort and distortion occur. Increasing sophistication of amplifier circuitry has gone some way to overcome this difficulty, providing such features as 'automatic gain control', or 'peak clipping' in which the peaks of sound are removed. The 'low frequency cut' introduced by selecting the 'H' position on the tone control is often helpful in reducing background noise and improving speech intelligibility.

Earphones

Earphones for body-worn aids are circular, and interchangeable, although it is important to use an earphone compatible with the rest of the aid. The low frequency response of insert earphones will usually go down to 20 Hz but the high frequency response seldom exceeds 5000 Hz. Earphones for ear-level aids have a more limited low frequency range but a better high frequency response.

Bone conduction aids

These have a vibrator in place of an earphone. This has a much more limited low and high frequency response and consumes much more power. Firm pressure against the sides of the head is necessary and this is often the cause of much discomfort. Such pressure may be achieved by an 'Alice band' spring over the head, or by strongly sprung spectacle frames. Bone conduction aids are much less widely used than conventional ear conduction aids, and find their chief application where an intractible tendency to infection and discharge precludes the wearing of an insert in the external meatus.

Batteries (more correctly, 'cells')

Three types are commonly used for body worn aids.
1. Zinc carbon.
2. Manganese alkaline.
3. Mercury.

The zinc carbon cells give the highest voltage initially, but rapidly deteriorate. The mercury cell gives a much more sustained voltage, and generally lasts over 2.5 times as long. The performance of the manganese alkaline cell lies intermediate between the two.

The suitability of zinc air batteries is being examined. These have almost twice the capacity of the corresponding mercury cell and contain considerably less mercury (thus reducing the problems of waste disposal). For head worn aids the mercury cell is most widely used. An alternative is the silver oxide cell which operates at 1.5 volts as compared with 1.35 volts from the mercury cell. This gives a small increase in output from the aid at the expense of much shorter batterly life.

Rechargable (nickel cadmium or silver zinc) batteries are available for all hearing aids. They have a performance similar to mercury cells and can be recharged for several years. They can represent a considerable economy but have not come into general use, presumably because of organisational difficulties.

With most aids there is no significant variation in battery consumption with different volume control settings: a steady current is consumed regardless of output. New NHS ear-level batteries are only issued against return of spent cells which are forwarded to Bristol Stores for proper disposal.

Inserts (or 'ear moulds')

Inserts are generally made of hard or soft acrylic from impressions taken with soft material similar to that used by dentists. The audiometrician takes the impression and posts it to the insert factory, which returns the finished insert 1 or 2 weeks later.

The patient then re-attends the hearing aid centre where the insert is checked to ensure that it is comfortable for the wearer, whilst at the same time forming an accurate seal.

The insert serves to hold the earphone in place and to seal the meatus thereby preventing acoustic feedback ('whistling'). Inserts may be 'ventilated' by drilling a narrow hole. This allows dissipation of lower frequencies and may be helpful for patients with a high tone loss. It may also lessen the tendency for otitis externa to develop in the occluded meatus.

Some patients appear to develop an idiosyncrasy to acrylic, with resulting otitis externa. An insert made of alternative material, such as vulcanite, may overcome this difficulty.

CROS hearing aids

Where a patient is severely deaf in one ear, it is possible to arrange an aid so that the microphone is on the deaf side. Sounds are conveyed across to the 'good' side to be fed into the ear via an open mould which does not affect the normal hearing on this side. Such a system, contralateral routing of signals (CROS), is most conveniently based on a spectacles frame. If hearing on the 'better' side is also impaired, an aid on this side may be incorporated into the CROS system. (CROS aids are not available through normal NHS sources).

Speaking tubes

Where hearing loss is only moderate at speech frequencies, old fashioned speaking tubes still have a place, and they may sometimes be surprisingly helpful even for the very deaf. They provide a gain of about 20 dB. If the speaker puts his mouth close to the tube, the sound enters the listener's ear at 90–100 dB.

Prescribing a hearing aid

Consideration of the patient's general condition and motivation, and examination of his ear, and of his audiogram, may give some guide as to whether the wearing of an aid will be successful, and as to which type is likely to be most suitable. Predictions are however by no means as dependable as is the case, for example, in refraction for spectacles. Trial with an aid, and of alternative models, is often necessary before the best results are obtained. Distortion tends to become a serious disadvantage as the maximum output of an aid is approached. It is therefore usually best to supply an aid providing adequate gain with the volume control turned halfway down.

Where both ears are equally deaf it may be best to fit two aids, one for each ear. When hearing loss is unequal on the two sides it may still be best to use two aids. If only one aid is to be provided. then if the better ear has useful unaided hearing the deafer ear will usually be fitted with an aid, whilst if neither ear has useful unaided hearing, it will be preferable to fit the aid in the better ear.

Coping with a hearing aid

Many patients using hearing aids encounter few difficulties.

For others however the aid is only partially satisfactory. Despite all efforts, distortion is likely to be a particular problem in the sensory and cochlear conductive forms of presbycusis, in which the audiogram is 'ski-slope' shaped. If the patient is unable to achieve at least 50% word discrimination he is likely to discard the aid.

Some aid users recognise from a change in tone that a battery is beginning to fail. On other occasions batteries may suddenly fail. If kept in a cool dry place spare batteries keep well, losing only an insignificant amount of charge. An adequate reserve supply should therefore always be at hand.

Leads on body aids tend to break after a few weeks so one or two should be held in reserve.

Wax tends to be pushed into the ear by the insert, and the general practitioner can render aid-using patients a valuable service by inspecting the ears and removing accumulated wax periodically.

It is desirable that the families of patients deaf enough to require an aid should understand that they are likely to be in difficulties, despite amplification. During conversation with a deaf person, the speaker should use a normal voice, and speak as distinctly as possible. He should position himself away from the glare of a window or light, so that his face is clearly visible, and should look at the patient, since visual clues from the eyes may facilitate communication.

Devices In The Home

Hearing aid users with severe hearing loss may be unable to follow television unless the set is turned up a good deal too loudly for the comfort of those with normal hearing.

This problem may be simply overcome by use of an induction lead plugged into the set and placed against the aid microphone. The signal is thereby induced in the aid without intervening conversion to sound waves and re-conversion to electromagnetic waves after attenuation across the room. Much improved sound reception is thereby achieved, and the aid user can regulate volume using the control on his aid. Small portable television sets are usually supplied with suitable sockets for an induction loop: in other cases the help of a television engineer may be required to fit a socket. The aid control must be switched to the T position.

For the less severely deaf, direct amplification with an independant microphone–amplifier–earphone system gives excellent results. Telephones may be fitted with a volume control for the convenience of the hard of hearing. British Telecom will fit an induction loop, on request, to standard telephones, enabling the hearing aid user to receive signals with the T position selected. All motorway emergency telephones have now been fitted with this modification. For patients who are unable to hear the telephone ringing, British Telecom can provide extension bells, or buzzers, hooters or flashing lights.

Deaf people may have difficulty in hearing the front door bell. The bell can alternatively be connected to the lighting systems so that during the daytime the lights come on, and at night the lights are diminished when the front door button is pressed. Sometimes flicker on the television screen is sufficient to draw a deaf person's attention to the ringing of the doorbell.

New television developments are proving of great help to the very deaf. Teletext enables viewers to receive written information on the screen from Ceefax (BBC) and Oracle (ITV), and increasing numbers of programmes are being sub-titled. Oracle offers information on deaf societies as well as instruction in lip reading. At British Telecom, research is underway on a device which will enable deaf people to hold telephone 'conversations'. Spoken words transmitted by telephone will be fed through a computer to appear in print on the Prestel screen.

Hearing dogs for the deaf

In the U.S.A. over 200 dogs have been specially trained to respond to household sounds (alarm clocks, door bells, dropped keys, whistling kettles, etc.) by attracting their severely deaf owner's attention and leading him in the appropriate direction. The contribution of these dogs in terms of companionship and affection may be of even greater importance than the purely practical assistance, invaluable though this is. In the U.K. this year a pilot scheme, the 'Hearing Dogs for the Deaf' programme, sponsored by the Royal National Institute for the Deaf, has been initiated (Fogle & Radcliffe, 1983). Dogs between 8 and 24 months old, usually chosen from homes for strays, are given a 4-month training in a home-like environment then introduced to the home of a severely or profoundly deaf person. A 'placement officer' working with the dog and new owner is provided for the first 10 days to consolidate the training.

Lip reading

Lip reading becomes increasingly important as deafness increases. Special instruction may be most beneficial, and is better provided early rather than late.

Much support is available from attendance at hard of hearing social groups-addresses of local organisations may be obtained from the RNID.

Organisations

Where recent onset of severe deafness is imposing serious strains within a family, the *Link Centre* in Sussex (The Centre for Deafened People, 19 Hartfield Road, Eastbourne, East Sussex BN21 2AX, telephone Eastbourne 22744) is invaluable, providing residential accommodation for the patient and his spouse for intensive rehabilitation.

The Royal National Institute for the Deaf, 105 Gower Street, London W1 1E (telephone 01–387–8033) is always willing to supply advice on all problems affecting deaf people , and provides a bimonthly publication called *Hearing*. For children the *National Deaf Childrens Society* can be contacted at 31 Gloucester Place, London W1H 4EA (telephone 01–486–3521/2). This society publishes a quarterly magazine called *Talk*.

Additional bodies include the following:

British Association of the Hard of Hearing, 7–11, Armstrong Road, London W3 7JL (Telephone 01–743–1110).

British Deaf Association, 38 Victoria Place, Carlisle CA1 5EX.

Greater London Association for the Disabled, 1 Thorpe Close, London W10 5XL publishes a useful information sheet 'Communication Aids for Deaf and Hard of Hearing People'.

Hearing Aid Industry Association, Broadway House, The Broadway, Wimbledon, London SW19 will advise on suppliers of hearing aids and will take up complaints from the public.

The Hard-of-Hearing Medical Society can give valuable advice to deaf doctors and their colleagues. Contact Dr Colin Green, 51 Croftdown Road, Harborne, Birmingham B178RE.

TINNITUS

Definition

Tinnitus may be defined as the sensation of a sound experienced where there is no external source. It is an extremely common symptom. A recent epidemiological study of four urban populations by the Institute of Hearing Research (1981) revealed that 17% of the general population suffer from significant tinnitus lasting more than 5–10 minutes.

Onset is most commonly in the sixth decade, but all age groups are affected. A study of 2000 school children in New York (Nodar, 1972) revealed a 13% incidence in normal children, rising to 59% in those who had failed screening tests for hearing. Most, but not all, cases of tinnitus suffer from some degree of hearing loss. Conversely, about 85% of patients with any hearing impairment have tinnitus (House, 1981). Most healthy people become aware of tinnitus when enclosed in a sound-proof room.

Two types of tinnitus have traditionally been recognised; objective, in which an identifiable source of sound exists in the head; and a much larger subjective (or 'idiopathic') group in which no source of sound is believed to be present.

Causes of objective tinnitus include the following:

1. Vascular bruit

(a) A regular pulsation synchronous with the heartbeat may be encountered during exertion in healthy individuals, and at rest in atherosclerotic patients.

(b) A distressing continuous roar may occur in the presence of arteriovenous fistulae, aneurysms, and other vascular malformations.

Vascular tinnitus may be audible to an examiner applying a stethoscope to the patient's head or neck.

2. Muscle clonus

Some patients experience bouts of 'clicking' tinnitus originating from myoclonic contractions of the tensor tympani, stapedius, or palatine muscles. Such tinnitus should be audible to an examiner listening through a tube inserted into the patient's external meatus.

3. Respiratory tinnitus

In some patients the Eustachian tube is unduly wide and patulous, and the sound of breath passing the orifice is plainly audible.

4. Cochlear tinnitus

In addition to afferent fibres in the cochlear nerve conveying impulses centrally, a small number of efferent fibres, of uncertain function, have been demonstrated (p. 68).

Using an extremely sensitive microphone, Kemp (1978) detected sounds in the ear, apparently generated by the cochlea. Possibly this sound generation is stimulated by discharge of 8th nerve efferent fibres. In some cases the frequency of sounds detected have coincided with the reported pitch of tinnitus.

This discovery has undermined the conventional classification of tinnitus into objective and subjective types, since a substantial but indeterminate portion of cases must now be transferred to the objective group.

Tinnitus may be very severe even after destruction of the labyrinth and section of the 8th nerve. In such circumstances the site of origin of the tinnitus must lie within the brain. Mechanisms for production of such 'central tinnitus' remain obscure.

Clinical features

Patients with tinnitus tend to belong to older age groups, and to be depressed. Most are also afflicted by some degree of deafness. The extent to which tinnitus interferes with everyday life seems largely to depend on individual personality. The more outgoing well organised person will treat the symptom as an annoyance. At the other end of the personality spectrum, tinnitus may come to dominate the patient's life.

Investigation

Tinnitus is so common, and so often innocuous, that full investigation is neither practicable nor desirable for most cases.

All patients troubled sufficiently to consult their doctor should be questioned regarding general health, and exposure to loud noise or ototoxic drugs. Examination should include inspection of the tympanic membranes, a simple hearing test using a whisper at 1 m, and auscultation of the head and neck with a stethoscope. The blood pressure should be recorded. An audiogram is helpful if only to document present hearing status for future reference.

Cases of unilateral tinnitus accompanied by deafness and/or vertigo require further investigation including audiometry, caloric testing, radiology, and possibly evoked response studies to exclude acoustic neuroma.

Management

Where a cause for tinnitus can be identified, specific measures are sometimes available.

1. Treatment of hypertension may attenuate tinnitus of vascular origin.
2. Where Menière's disease underlies tinnitus, betahistine appears the most effective drug.
3. Tinnitus arising as a result of otosclerotic stapes fixation or acoustic neuroma may improve following surgery.
4. Tinnitus arising from syphilitic cochlear involvement may improve after therapy with penicillin combined with steroids.
5. In one small group of cases, pulsatile tinnitus is relieved by light pressure on the jugular vein. Such patients are said to be permanently cured by ligation of the internal and external jugular vein on the affected side.
6. Myoclonic tinnitus has been successfully treated with carbamazepine.
7. In tinnitus arising from respiratory airflow in cases of patulous Eustachian tubes, success has attended both cauterisation of the tube with silver nitrate to cause stenosis, and injection of silicone material round the orifice.

The great majority patients with tinnitus, despite modern advances in investigation, belong to the 'subjective' category, for whom no specific treatment is available.

The best results are achieved where good rapport exists between patient and doctor. The sufferer needs reassurance that his complaint is understood, and that it is a common problem, an inconvenience rather than a disease, and that no drug is likely to be of much assistance.

Although local anaesthetics administered intravenously relieve tinnitus, the effect is only short lived and no dependable oral agent has yet emerged.

Struck by the comment of one sufferer that he could not hear his tinnitus whilst standing beside a fountain, Vernon in the USA in 1977 introduced a 'masker' worn like a post-aural hearing aid. The device enabled the user to 'drown' his own tinnitus by means of a noise he could control himself. For some cases the masker and a hearing aid have been combined in one unit.

Maskers are available in ENT departments in the UK and are appropriate for more disturbed patients. Many users report that intermittent use of a masker relieves for long periods a distressing tinnitus which was previously incessant.

Some patients are unaware of their tinnitus during the working day, but are troubled on reaching the quiet of the bedroom at night, and cannot sleep. They may be helped by a radio (with or without an earpiece) arranged to switch itself off once they are asleep.

The patient relieved of his tinnitus by the cascade of a fountain (Dr Charles Unice) went on to found the American Tinnitus Association. In the UK, Mr Jack Ashley MP launched the British Tinnitus Association in July 1979, under the aegis of the Royal National Institute for the Deaf, 105 Gower Street, London WC1E 6AH. Distressed patients should be encouraged to contact the Association, which issues a quarterly newsletter giving information about local patient-support groups, research advances, and answers to patients' letters.

DIZZINESS AND VERTIGO

Mechanism of balance

The labyrinth responds to alteration in angular velocity (semi-circular canals) and to alteration in direction of gravity and linear acceleration (utricle and, possibly, saccule). The method by which these changes are sensed involves deflection of 'hairs' of the hair cells. Each hair cell has 50–110 stereocilia, and one 'kinocilium' which lies at the periphery of the stereocilia. Displacement of stereocilia towards the kinocilium results in depolarisation, whilst displacement away from the kinocilium leads to hyperpolarisation. In the semicircular canals the hair cells in the ampulla of the lateral canal are positioned with their kinocilia on the utricular side, whilst in the ampullae of the other two canals the kinocilia are on the side to the cell remote from the utricle.

The macula of the utricle (Fig. 5.17) is divided into two zones by a curved line (striola), all the kinocilia being on the side of the hair cells towards the line. The saccular macule is divided by a line, all the kinocilia lying on the side of the hair cells away from the line. On account of the curves of the demarcation lines (almost semi-

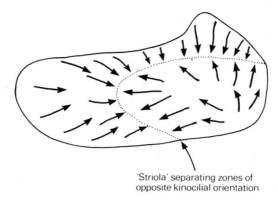

'Striola' separating zones of opposite kinocilial orientation

Fig. 5.17. Schematic representation of utricular macule with respect to position of Kinocilium.

circles) various positions of the head in space selectively maximally affect different parts of the maculae.

Animal experiments have demonstrated that at rest there is a steady discharge rate of action potentials in the vestibular nerve. If the lateral canal is opened and connected to a pump, positive pressure causes head and eye movements to the opposite side, and negative pressure the reverse. These phenomena are accompanied by increases or decreases respectively in vestibular nerve action potential discharge rates.

The association of changing nerve action potential discharge rates with alterations in head position has been clearly established in the case of the utricular macule. Although structurally the saccular macule appears complementary to the utricular macule, experimental confirmation of an equilibrium function is lacking, and in lower animals it appears sensitive to low frequency sound vibrations.

Central connections

Each vestibular nerve conveys about 20 000 afferent fibres, and also about 200 efferent fibres, distributed to all cristae and maculae. The function of the efferent fibres remains unclear, but it is suggested they provide 'negative feedback control', analogous to disconnecting a number of incoming lines on a hospital telephone switchboard to avoid overloading it in the event of a major disaster.

The central connections of the vestibular pathway are extremely complex, but have the effect of co-ordinating information from the vestibule, eye, cerebellum, reticular formation, and spinal cord through the vestibular nuclei in the upper medulla. Vestibular information reaches the cortex and is involved with conscious orientation in space. The cortex is however not concerned with eye movement co-ordination.

Vertigo

Although no sharp distinction can be made between the symptoms of dizziness and vertigo, dizziness is generally a milder symptom, a positional insecurity or unsteadiness, which may result from a wide variety of general causes. Vertigo is usually a more dramatic symptom, involving a sensation of rotation. either of the subject or his surroundings. It occurs when information from the vestibular apparatus conflicts with that received from the eyes, proprioceptive receptors in muscles, tendons and joints, and touch receptors, particularly in the soles of the feet. The cause of vertigo may be central, involving the 8th nerve or its central connections, or peripheral, in the vestibular apparatus.

Clues as to whether vertigo is of central or peripheral origin may be obtained from the history.

Central vertigo

In vertigo of *central* origin:
Hallucinations of movement are generally less evident
Onset is slow
Intensity is seldom severe
Duration is generally long (maybe several weeks)
Head position usually is irrelevant
Nausea and vomiting are mild or absent
Tinnitus and deafness are unusual
Disturbances of consciousness and abnormal neurological signs are common.

Causes of central vertigo. These include vertebrobasilar insufficiency, multiple sclerosis, acoustic neuroma, cerebral tumours, head injury, and epilepsy.

Peripherally produced vertigo

In *peripherally* produced vertigo there is usually:
A hallucination of movement
Sudden onset

Severe intensity
Short duration
Head position usually affects the severity of the vertigo
Nystagmus is virtually always present
Nausea and vomiting, tinnitus and deafness are frequent accompaniments
Consciousness is usually well preserved

Causes of peripheral vertigo. These include Menière's Disease (p. 91), sudden vestibular failure, benign paroxysmal positional vertigo, labyrinthine involvement in the presence of middle ear disease, otosclerosis, or from ototoxic drugs or trauma.

Sudden vestibular failure

Also known as 'vestibular neuronitis' 'epidemic vertigo' or 'acute labyrinthitis', this condition results in sudden loss of vestibular function on one side, usually with no disturbance of hearing.

There is violent vertigo, nausea and vomiting and prostration. Any movement of the head exacerbates the symptoms. The condition slowly subsides so that by the fourth day the patient can usually begin to move about very cautiously in the room, changing the position of his head as little as possible and holding onto furniture. Balance gradually returns over the course of about 3 weeks, but instability when over-tired or in the dark may last longer. Recovery is eventually complete and there is no tendency to recurrence.

The condition is common. Brill (1982) was able to study 50 cases in his 8200 patient group practice between 1976 and 1979. He confirmed a viral cause in 28%: mostly Influenza A virus, and gives reasons for suspecting that in many cases as yet unidentified viruses may be responsible. 25% of his patients were pyrexial. Head injury, labyrinthine end artery obstruction, multiple sclerosis, diabetic neuropathy, and brain stem encephalitis may also cause acute vestibular failure.

Nystagmus is usually present in the early stages (50% in Brill's series by the time he saw them). For the first few days it is '3rd degree' (present on looking forward and to either side), with the quick component towards the healthy side. Nystagmus reduces to 1st degree (present only when looking in the direction of the fast component) before disappearing.

Treatment. In the early stages the patient is understandably very alarmed. Intramuscular prochlorperazine 12.5 mg or chlorpromazine 50 mg gives symptomatic relief but may need to be repeated during the first 2–3 days until a 'labyrinthine sedative' such as cinnarizine 15 mg three times 1 day can be taken orally. This should be continued for at least 3 weeks, until the sense of equilibrium is fully restored.

It is very helpful to the patient and his relatives if they are prepared at the outset for the likely duration of the disability.

Benign paroxysmal posterial vertigo

In this condition short-lived vertigo (measured in seconds) occurs whenever the head is placed in a particular position. It typically occurs at night when turning over in bed.

The cause is believed to be detachment of mineral particles from the otolith organ in the utricle. These fall into the ampulla of the posterior semicircular canal under the influence of gravity when the head is placed in the appropriate position, and exert pressure on the cupola, giving rise to a temporary sensation of rotation.

A preceding viral infection, head injury, or degenerative changes may be responsible for the detachment. Symptoms usually continue for weeks or a few months, then cease.

The diagnosis, indicated by the history, can be confirmed by positional tests.

Positional tests

The patient is asked to sit upright on the couch, facing forwards, and is then gently laid back with his head straight. He is asked to look at the examiner's forehead. Any nystagmus is noted. After lying back for a few seconds, he is asked to sit upright again, and again nystagmus is looked for (Fig. 5.18).

The patient is then asked to turn his head to one side, and with the examiner holding his head he is again laid back; the head still deviated. After a short pause vertigo and nystagmus may occur. If there is no response the patient is sat upright again, and any nystagmus noted. The examiner then moves to the other side of the couch and the tests are repeated with the patient's head turned to this side. If no vertigo and nystagmus are provoked in any of the three directions, lying down or on returning to the upright position, the test is negative and the diagnosis in doubt.

A positive response occurs when, after a pause with the head laid in one position or another, vertigo and nystagmus develop, and persist

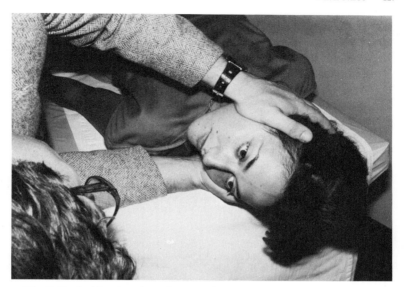

Fig. 5.18. Positional testing: observing for nystagmus.

for some 10–15 seconds. The nystagmus is characteristically rotatory, beating towards the downwards ear. There may be short-lived 'rebound' vertigo and nystagmus when the patient sits up. If the head is again laid into the provoking position, vertigo and nystagmus recur but with less severity and shorter duration. Further testing without a rest period yields dwindling and finally absent responses.

The features of a few seconds' latency, short duration, and fatiguability, distinguish labyrinthine positional vertigo from the rare positional vertigo of central origin (where nystagmus is instant in onset, enduring so long as the head remains in the position concerned, and not fatiguable).

Treatment consists of explanation, reassurance regarding the good prognosis, and advice regarding avoidance of the provocative head positions.

REFERENCES

Beales P H 1981 in Otosclerosis. John Wright & Sons, Bristol, p. 83
Brill G C 1982 Acute Labyrinthitis: a possible association with influenze. Journal of the Royal College of General Practitioners 32: 47–50
Fogle B, Radcliffe A 1983 Hearing dogs for the deaf. The Practitioner 227:1051
Fuller A P 1967 Personal communication

Hof E 1976 Meningitis und Labyrinthitis im Kindesalter. Otorhinolaryngology 38 (Suppl 1): 25–31
House J W 1981 In: Tinnitus, p. 33. CIBA Foundation Symposium 85. Pitman Books Ltd, London
Kemp D T 1978 Stimulated acoustic emissions from within the human auditory system. Journal of the Acoustic Society of America 64:1386
Matsunaga T 1976 Otolaryngology (Tokyo) 48:65
Morrison A W 1967 Genetic factors in otosclerosis. Annals of the Royal College of Surgeons of England 41: 202–237
Morrison A W 1969 Management of severe deafness in adults. The otologist's contribution. Proceedings of the Royal Society of Medicine 62: 959–965
Morrison A W 1975 in management of sensorineural deafness Butterworths London
Nodar R H 1972 Tinnitus aurium in school age children, a survey. Journal of Auditory Research 12: 133–135
Philipzoon A J 1962 Journal of Laryngology 76: 593
Pulec J L 1977 Indications for surgery in Menière's disease. Laryngoscope. 87 4 (Pt 1): 542–556
Rosen S, Plester D, El-Mofty A, Rosen H 1964 Archives of Otolaryngology 79:34
Shambaugh G H Jr, Causse J 1974 Ten years experience with fluoride in otosclerotic (otospongiotic) patients. Annals of Otology 83:635
Shea J J, Emmett J R 1981 The medical treatment of tinnitus. Journal of Laryngology and Ototoly. (Suppl 4):130
Stahle J, Stahle C, Arenberg I K 1978 Incidence of Menière's Disease. Archives of Otolaryngology 104: 99–102
Taylor I G 1980 The prevention of sensorineural deafness Journal of Laryngology and Otology 94: 1327–1347
Thomsen J, Bretlau P, Tos M, Johnsen N J 1981 Placebo effect in surgery for Menière's disease. Archives of Otolaryngology 107: 271–277
Westmore G A Fuersden I D 1981 Noise induced hearing loss and orchestral musicians. Achives of Otolaryngology 107: 761–764

Part 3
The Nose

6.

Anatomy and Examination of the Nose

The nose and nasopharynx constitute a filter and air conditioner for protection of the lungs, and local immune mechanisms are at the 'front line' in combating air-borne pathogens.

The *nasal cavity* bears on its lateral wall (Fig. 6.1) three mucosa-covered bony *turbinates*: superior, middle and inferior, arranged like shelves one above the other with their free edges turned downwards. The superior turbinate is usually too high up to be seen

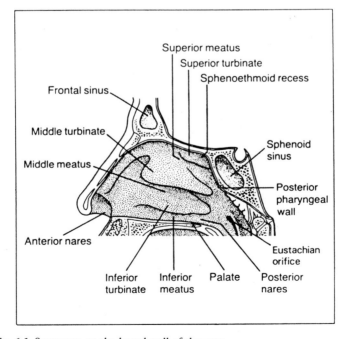

Fig. 6.1 Structures on the lateral wall of the nose.

through the anterior nares. The turbinates form the roofs of three *'meati'*: superior, middle and inferior. The spheno-ethmoid recess lies above and behind the superior meatus.

Sinuses

The sphenoid sinus opens into the spheno-ethmoid recess, and the posterior ethmoid air cells into the superior meatus, whilst the anterior and middle ethmoid air cells, frontal and maxillary sinuses, all open into the middle meatus. The Eustachian tube, bony in its posterior one-third and supported by cartilage in its anterior two-thirds, opens into the nasopharynx behind the nasal cavity.

Except in the nasal vestibule, where the epithelium is squamous and hairs are present, the nasal cavity and sinuses are lined by ciliated columnar epithelium bearing mucus secreting cells and goblet cells. The sub-mucosal tissue is loose, highly vascular, and contains many glands and, especially in children, numerous small aggregations of lymphoid tissue.

The mucociliary system

Since the upper respiratory tract incorporates several 'dead end' chambers (including the sinuses and middle ear cavities) an effective clearance mechanism is essential for removal of cellular remnants, atmospheric contaminants, bacteria and other debris. This is provided by the fundamentally important mucociliary system. Ciliated cells are present in all members of the animal kingdom (except, it appears, flatworms) and in mammals serve the function of mucus transport (and, as spermatozoa tails, sperm transport). Respiratory tract epithelial cells carry 250–300 cilia/cell, about 8 μm long and 0.1–0.2 μm wide. All cilia have a similar structure on cross section (Fig. 6.2): nine double tubes surrounding two single tubes. The making and breaking of bridges between the tubes lead them to slide in relation to one another causing the cilia to 'beat'. The tubes are composed of the protein tubulin, whilst the intertubular bridges are formed from another protein, dynein. Cilia cannot function without dynein, and this has been found absent in patients with Kartagener's syndrome (sinusitis, bronchitis and dextrocardia) leading to recurrent sinusitis, otitis media, bronchitis, and infertility.

The direction of beating of cilia is determined in early embryonic life and never changes. Human cilia beat at 500–1000 strokes/min,

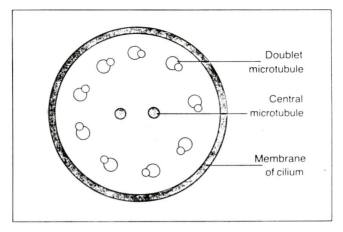

Fig. 6.2 Cross section of a cilium.

and shift the mucus blanket at a rate of 11–16 mm/min. Such is the strength of the combined and co-ordinated ciliary beating that a piece of excised frog's gullet, laid faced downwards on a moist glass rod held horizontally, will travel from one end to the other.

For ciliary action to function effectively the composition of the interciliary fluid, and of the overlying mucus blanket, is crucial. No molecules big enough to get between the cilia and interfere with their movement must be present. Mucus elaborated in the Golgi apparatus of the goblet cells is secreted to form a thin mucus 'blanket' (Fig 6.3) on which particles for clearance are carried along, as

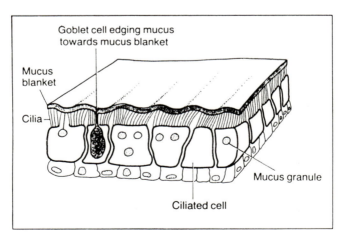

Fig. 6.3 The ciliary-mucus blanket system.

if on a conveyor belt, continually shifted by the co-ordinated beating of the underlying cilia. The physical properties of the mucus are critical: the component molecules must be cross-linked for the blanket to 'cohere together'. If the mucus layer is broken down (for example by treatment with DDT) the clearance function ceases although the cilia continue to beat. The cross-linkage is sometimes excessive (as in the 'glue' of glue ear) or inadequate (as in the serous fluid of serous otitis media). Oxygen and carbon dioxide concentration and pH are amongst the factors known to influence both ciliary action and mucus cross-linkage.

Examination of the nose

Anterior rhinoscopy

The inside of childrens' noses is often conveniently examined merely by pressing the tip upwards, and inspecting the nasal cavities with the help of a torch, or head mirror.

For adults a Thudichum's speculum is usually required to open up the nasal vestibule (an aural speculum may be used but is less satisfactory). When about to have their noses examined, patients tend to tilt their heads backwards in an effort to be helpful. This of course puts most of the nasal cavity out of view and the head must be restored to a vertical position. The speculum must be held very gently, and when purchasing a Thudichum's speculum care should be taken that the spring in the handle is weak or nonexistent: strong springs can be difficult to control and cause pain.

It is often necessary to shrink the nasal mucosa in order to examine the posterior parts of the nasal cavities. A 10% cocaine spray is convenient for this purpose, since it causes rapid decongestion and surface anaesthesia, allowing introduction of instruments if necessary. Alternatively, 1% ephedrine nose drops may be used.

In order to carry out a visual 'sweep' of the nasal cavities, the position of the patient's head must be adjusted several times. Use of a head mirror frees both hands, one on top of the patient's head to control the position whilst the other holds the speculum. As with the contents of any dark chamber, much better results are obtained in a darkened or shaded part of the consulting room.

Posterior rhinoscopy

The patient is asked to open his mouth wide. With the tongue lowered using a tongue depressor, a small mirror is introduced behind the edge of the soft palate. By adjusting the position of the mirror, the posterior edge of the nasal septum, the posterior ends of the turbinates, any adenoids present, and sometimes the Eustachian openings can be seen. Satisfactory mirror examination of the post-nasal space is not possible in all patients, even in expert hands. Fibroptic endoscopy, or direct examination under anaesthesia in hospital, may be necessary.

Assessment of nasal deviation

After nasal injury, the severity of lateral deviation may be difficult to gauge from the front. A better idea may be obtained by looking down the patient's head from above, when any deviation will be more easily appreciated.

7

Upper respiratory tract infections

CORYZA

This is possibly the commonest viral infection in man. The average young adult has been held to have seven colds annually (Hope Simpson, 1958). The epithelium of the nasal cavity, sinuses and nasopharynx is most commonly involved, but infection may extend to the lower respiratory tract. Involvement of the epiglottis, larynx or trachea may cause life-threatening obstruction in infants and young children.

Children are particularly prone to colds, chiefly because they have not yet developed specific immunity to virus types. They frequently harbour viruses and constitute a hazard to bronchitic adults. The particular susceptibility of school teachers to upper respiratory tract infections is a common observation in general practice.

The frequency of colds is remarkably constant throughout the world, with the exception of the arctic and antarctic regions. Colds due to rhinoviruses occur all the year round, with peaks in spring and autumn, whilst colds due to coronaviruses occur most frequently between December and March. Several different viruses are circulating in the community, and even within a family, at any one time.

The influence of environment on transmission of colds is uncertain. Cross infection appears less common in conditions of optimal humidity, warmth and ventilation. 'Chilling' is widely believed to lead to 'catching cold' but this has not been experimentally confirmed (Andrewes, 1975). Malnutrition and chronic infection lower resistance to colds. Viruses causing common colds are ubiquitous, and development of a cold must be attributable either to lowered resistance or to exposure to overwhelming infection.

An intact muco-ciliary system is essential to the health of the upper respiratory tract. Pronounced septal deviations, polypi, hypertrophied turbinates, and scars and adhesions in the nose, from past injuries or surgery, can all interfere with the movement of the blanket and increase the frequency and severity of colds.

Causative viruses

The chief viruses causing colds are:

1. Rhinoviruses
2. Adenoviruses
3. Para-influenzal viruses
4. Respiratory syncitial viruses
5. Coronaviruses
6. Enteroviruses (especially coxsackie viruses and echoviruses)

Colds due to the adenoviruses are often associated with pharyngitis and conjunctivitis. Para-influenzal and respiratory syncitial viruses frequently invade the lower respiratory tract, especially in infants and young children.

Rhinoviruses

These are the commonest cause of colds, responsible for about a half of all cases. Incubation period is 2–4 days, and the duration is less than 1 week but sometimes up to 2 weeks. More than 100 serotypes are known and several may be circulating at one time, repeated infections in the same patient developing despite the raising of neutralising antibodies specific for each type in turn.

Cross-infection occurs by air-borne droplet transmission and from the fingers of patients and handled objects.

Adenoviruses

These cause outbreaks of colds in crowded communities. Endemic infection in the general population probably causes less than 5% of colds. One strain (type 8) is also responsible for epidemic kerato-conjunctivitis, and outbreaks of this have been traced to contaminated instruments in hospital eye clinics. As well as acute coryza, adenoviruses can cause chronic infection, and can be isolated from 50–90% of tonsils and adenoids removed (Zaiman et al, 1955). There are 33 serological types.

Para-influenzal viruses

In addition to causing febrile colds with sore throat and cough in adults, para-influenzal viruses may cause dangerous laryngo-tracheo-bronchitis in infants. There are four serological types. Type one outbreaks tend to occur in alternate years. Type three shows a predilection for younger children, and outbreaks occur annually.

Respiratory syncitial viruses (RSV)

In addition to causing colds in adults, RSV infection leads to serious bronchiolitis and pneumonia in infants under 1 year old, carrying a mortality of up to 5%. Outbreaks occur each winter.

Coronaviruses

These cause some 20% of common colds. There are at least three antigenic types.

Enteroviruses (including polio-myelitis viruses, coxsackie and echoviruses)

Characteristically, enteroviruses enter the body through the mouth, invade the lymphoid tissue of the alimentary tract (including the pharynx) and set up a viraemia.

Some enteroviruses however, particularly coxsackie A21 and B3 and echoviruses types 11 and 20, can cause typical colds.

Influenza

Influenza viruses groups A, B and C can all cause rhinitis resembling the common cold, but this is generally overshadowed by pulmonary, gastro-intestinal, or general symptoms.

Clinical picture of coryza

Four stages may be recognised.

1. Prodromal, lasting a few hours. Local invasion causes a hot, dry, tickling sensation of the throat.
2. Early reaction. Infection spreads to adjacent mucous membranes. This stage lasts a few hours or days and, as infection spreads, the areas of mucous membrane first involved may have recovered. Sneezing, watery rhinorrhoea, nasal obstruction and soreness and dryness of the throat occur. The mucosa is red and swollen. Mild toxaemia and sometimes fever develop.
3. Secondary infection. After about 2 days rhinorrhoea thickens, diminishes, and becomes mucopurulent. Toxaemia increases.
4. Resolution occurs gradually and is generally complete after 5-10 days.

Complications

Some degree of pharyngitis is common during a cold. Sinusitis and acute otitis media are frequent complications of colds. Tonsilitis, laryngitis, tracheitis, and involvement of the lower respiratory tract and gastro-intestinal tract may all complicate colds.

Temporary anosmia commonly accompanies colds, oedematous mucosa in the vault of the nasal cavity isolating the olfactory epithelium. Some viruses, particularly of the influenza group, can damage the olfactory neural tissue, which becomes replaced by fibrous tissue. A characteristic of the resultant permanent anosmia is that patients describe a single very weak smell whatever the provoking odour. (Single non-discriminating response of Douek).

About one-third of all cases of sudden vestibular failure have upper respiratory infection. In a group of patients who developed sudden sensorineural hearing loss in the course of an upper respiratory infection, and who subsequently came to autopsy, severe atrophy of the hair cells of the organ of Corti was found (Schuknecht et al, 1973).

Rarely, distant toxic complications of colds occur including polyarthritis, skin rashes and nephritis.

Diagnosis

This is usually obvious from the history and general picture. There is no way of distinguishing the causative virus of a simple cold on clinical grounds, but the nature of any complications may suggest the identity of the virus concerned. Complement fixation tests may confirm this, but are of little more than academic interest.

Management

General

Until an effective antiviral agent becomes available, treatment can only be symptomatic. Most healthy people developing a cold try to disregard it and carry on as normally as possible. Some turn to aspirin, paracetamol, hot drinks, inhalations, oral and topical decongestants, large doses of vitamin C, whisky nightcaps, and other trusted remedies.

Care must be taken over the use of decongestants, both oral and topical, in the presence of cardiovascular disease. They may antagonise hypotensive drugs and severe reactions may occur in patients receiving monoamine oxidase inhibitor drugs.

Vitamin C is reputed to prevent or abort colds. Vitamin deficiency predisposes to infection, and mild vitamin C deficiency may not be very uncommon. A supplement for people at risk of deficiency, in a dose of 50mg/day, is desirable. Some have assumed that high doses of vitamin C in healthy people on adequate diets would have an antiviral effect. Several studies have been carried out in an endeavour to establish this claim, and even potentially toxic doses have been advocated. Most studies have given negative results and any benefit must be so small that it is not clinically useful (Tyrrell, 1981).

Antibiotics. These can have no effect on the course of the common cold, but may be justified as a prophylactic in those prone to complications such as otitis media, sinusitis, or chest infections. They may also be helpful where secondary bacterial rhinitis has developed, evidenced by yellowish or greenish nasal discharge. Penicillin and amoxycillin are widely used in children, and tetracylines in adults.

Interferon production is the chief natural defence mechanism during the acute phase of viral invasion. This protein is released from infected cells and, if taken up by unaffected cells, renders them resistant to viral infection. It is present in blood and tissues during acute viral infection and is probably responsible for recovery. The possibility of administering interferon produced in the laboratory is under exploration. Genetically produced interferon, being 99% pure, holds great promise.

ACUTE SINUSITIS

Description

Any of the sinuses may be infected, but the maxillary sinuses are of prime importance, being often alone involved, and seldom spared when other sinuses are infected. Sometimes all the sinuses are involved – pansinusitis. Sinusitis is an important cause of morbidity 500 000 working days were estimated by the DHSS to be lost as a result in 1971.

Sinus infection complicates about 0.5% of common colds (Dingle et al, 1964). Acute sinusitis leads to discomfort or pain over the sinuses and often referred to the distribution of nerves involved in the inflammation. There is usually anosmia, and often cacosmia, and nasal and/or postnasal discharge.

These local symptoms are often accompanied by general malaise, fever and headache. In some patients symptoms are mild, their persistence rather than severity suggesting the diagnosis.

Aetiology

Ten per cent of cases of maxillary sinusitis arise from spread of dental infection, either periapical abscess (the 1st and 2nd upper molars being most commonly involved) or periodontitis with spread of gum infection via the lymphatics. The layer of bone separating the tooth roots from the maxillary sinus cavity may be very thin in adults, and extraction of a tooth may open a route for entry of infection.

Otherwise, sinusitis is almost always a complication of upper respiratory tract infection. Obstruction of the maxillary ostium is presumably responsible. Drettner and Lindholm (1967) investigated patients with colds, introducing a needle connected to a manometer and wash bottle into the sinus. They demonstrated that, of 44 sinuses in patients with acute rhinitis, only eight had patent ostia. Sixteen had an obstruction which could be overcome by blowing or sniffing. The remaining 20 were completely obstructed.

Presumably infection has entered the sinus before blockage of the ostium, and failure of the mucociliary clearance system favours invasion of the sinus mucosa by viruses and bacteria, particularly anaerobic commensuals. Inflammatory hyperaemia, oedema, and exudate further obstruct the sinus ostium.

Contributory factors

Swimming with a cold, and especially diving, may lead to acute sinusitis. Pathogens in the water or chlorine, which may damage the mucociliary system, increase the risk. Poor general health, smoking, and bad housing conditions are associated with increased incidence of sinus infection. Malformations of the nose predispose to sinus infection: deviation of the nasal septum to one side, with compensatory hypertrophy of the middle turbinate on the other, may obstruct drainage from the maxillary, frontal, and ethmoid sinuses on both sides. Sinus drainage obstruction may occur in any form of rhinitis. Allergic rhinitis with nasal polypi is frequently associated with sinus infection.

Causative organisms

Viruses commonly playing an initial role in the development of acute sinusitis include:

1. Rhinoviruses
2. Parainfluenza viruses I and II
3. RSV
4. Echo 28
5. Coxsackie A21

Bacterial invasion follows, by *Strep. pneumoniae* or *Haemophilus influenzae* in over 50% of cases (Gwaltney et al, 1981). Anaerobic organisms, usually commensals in the upper respiratory tract, may become invasive pathogens in the presence of viral infection.

Diagnosis

Acute sinusitis is to be suspected when pain in the cheek or over the frontal area follows development of a head cold. Tenderness is often present over infected maxillary or frontal sinuses. Pain from infected ethmoids is deep seated behind the eyes and may be accompanied by tenderness at the back of the bridge of the nose, just below the inner canthus. Sphenoidal pain may be felt in the centre of the head radiating toward the back of the neck.

Inspection of the face may reveal puffiness over the frontal, maxillary, or ethmoidal sinuses.

Anterior rhinoscopy

This often reveals reddened swollen nasal mucosa, and yellow or greenish mucopus may be visible, emerging from the middle meatus if ostial obstruction is not yet complete.

Examination of the throat may disclose a mucopurulent postnasal drip.

Bacteriological examination

A nasal swab should ideally be taken for culture and sensitivities before chemotherapy begins, although it will not necessarily reflect the situation inside an obstructed sinus.

Transillumination

This may be helpful, demonstrating maxillary sinus opacity. It must be carried out in darkness: a broom cupboard is the traditional venue. The patient closes his lips round a bright pen torch held centrally in his mouth. Most help is obtained where there is a marked difference in brightness of illumination on the two sides. A fair degree of accuracy can be achieved, and confidence increases with familiarisation. This simple test is well worthwhile where X-rays are not readily available.

Radiology

Infected sinuses are radio-opaque (Fig. 7.1). Two postero-anterior views are often taken, one with the head 'erect' to show the ethmoid and frontal sinuses best, and one with the head tilted backwards, lowering the petrous temporal bones out of the line of view to show the maxillary sinuses best. A lateral skull view is needed to examine the sphenoid sinus.

Opacity of a sinus does not, of course, confirm the presence of infection: similar radiological appearances occur in allergic conditions, barotrauma, polypi, malignant disease, following sinus surgery, or in sinus agenesis.

Where the sinus contains fluid and air, X-rays may reveal a fluid level. If doubt exists, the presence of fluid may be confirmed by repeating the film with the head tilted to one side.

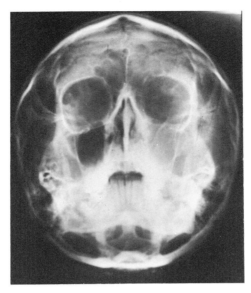

Fig. 7.1. Acute left maxillary sinusitis (Courtesy of Dept of Medical Illustration, St Bartholomew's Hospital, London)

Treatment

Treatment is essentially medical. Once well established, infection may be difficult to eradicate and increasing damage to the mucociliary system favours progression to chronic sinusitis. It is therefore highly desirable that the general practitioner should identify and treat acute sinusitis early, recognising that some patients may not complain of severe symptoms.

Antibiotics

A recently reported study (Gwaltney et al, 1981) of the effectiveness of ampicillin, amoxycillin, co-trimoxazole, and cefaclor in acute sinusitis showed all to be effective, and equally so.

Supportive treatment

Energetic efforts should be made to decongest the nasal and sinus mucosa in order to restore sinus drainage. Drops such as 1% ephedrine should be instilled into the nose, with the head tilted backwards, three or four times/day. Oral decongestants such as

Dimotapp LA tablets, one at night, are widely used. Aspirin or stronger analgesics may be needed. Steam inhalations medicated with volatile oils (as in Karvol capsules) are soothing and appear to promote drainage.

CHRONIC SINUSITIS

Aetiology

Chronic sinusitis can usually be recognised as the end result of incompletely resolved attacks of acute sinusitis. It may occasionally develop insidiously after a cold or dental infection. Aetiology is basically that of acute sinusitis: irreversible destruction of the mucociliary system results in chronic disease of the sinus mucosa.

Pathology

Three forms of mucosal change are recognised.

Polypoid sinusitis

Inflammatory changes affect mainly the efferent vessels. Lymphatics and soft tissues are secondarily affected. Recurring periphlebitis or perilymphangiitis results in fibrosis. Oedema, polypi, periosteal reaction and bone rarification may occur.

Atrophic sinusitis

Afferent vessels are mainly affected. There is cellular reaction round arterioles, with vessel wall thickening, lumen narrowing, and often endarteritis and thrombosis.

Both polypoid and atrophic sinusitis may develop at different places in the same sinus.

Papillary hypertrophic sinusitis

This is uncommon, but important since it may be confused with carcinoma at operation, until histology is available. There is metaplasia of epithelium to the stratified squamous form. Papillae develop infiltrated with inflammatory cells.

Clinical picture

Patients with chronic sinusitis usually complain of pain. This is sometimes labelled 'vacuum headache' in the belief that it originates as a result of blocked ostia with resultant creation of a partial vacuum. This is unlikely: negative pressure induced through a needle in the maxillary sinus does not cause pain (Drettner, 1967). Pain is probably the result of inflammation in the region of mucosal nerve endings.

Most patients with chronic sinusitis complain of nasal obstruction, often due to factors such as septal deviation responsible for the sinusitis.

Nasal discharge and post-nasal drip, often offensive, are common, often originating from associated rhinitis.

Epistaxis may occur. Disturbances of smell are common, including cacosmia (in which an unpleasant odour is noticeable to others as well as to the patient).

Chronic sinusitis may predispose to recurrent tonsillitis, pharyngitis, laryngitis, and otitis media. General health is undermined through toxic absorption.

Diagnosis

Anterior rhinoscopy may reveal structural abnormalities likely to cause sinus blockage, and the middle meatus should be examined for pus or polypi.

Posterior rhinoscopy may reveal pus in the nasopharynx, and antro-choanol polypi at the posterior nares.

Transillumination and radiology have been considered on page 145.

Antral puncture

Washout of the maxillary sinus via a cannula inserted through the lateral wall of the nose beneath the inferior turbinate serves both a diagnostic and therapeutic role in chronic sinusitis. It is a common out-patient procedure for adults, but for children admission for general anaesthesia is needed.

Bacteriological examination of washings may give useful information regarding infecting organisms and their antibiotic sensitivities. Washing away of infected material may be sufficient to permit resolution of infection, but sometimes repeated washouts are needed.

Management

Antral puncture and washout is an essential part of treatment in chronic sinusitis. Since individual general practitioners would be unlikely to carry out the procedure with sufficient frequency to maintain proficiency, patients with chronic sinusitis are referred to ENT departments for further management.

Conservative treatment, including repeated antral washouts, antibiotics and decongestants may allow chronic infection to resolve. Abnormalities underlying infection, such as septal deviations and polypi, may require attention.

For more persistent cases intranasal antrostomy, sometimes performed concurrently with correction of septal deviations, may improve sinus drainage sufficiently to permit resolution. Where problems continue, a Caldwell–Luc operation may be required. With the upper lip elevated, the front of the maxillary sinus is opened above the teeth. All diseased mucosa is curetted out, and a large intranasal antrostomy is fashioned.

Nowadays drainage operations on other sinuses are only rarely performed.

Complications

Complications of chronic sinusitis include the following.

1. Cellulitis, osteitis or osteomyelitis by direct extension of infection.
2. Mucocoele of the frontal sinus which may displace the eye downwards and outwards (Fig. 7.2).
3. Pyocoele.
4. Fistula, including:
    a. Fistula from the frontal or ethmoid sinuses, opening to the surface above the eye.
    b. Oro-antral fistula following dental extraction.
5. Intracranial spread may occur from frontal or ethmoid infection.
6. Cavernous sinus thrombosis is a very rare complication.

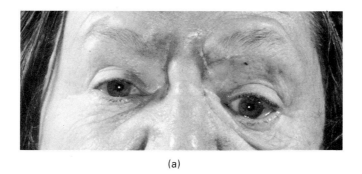
(a)

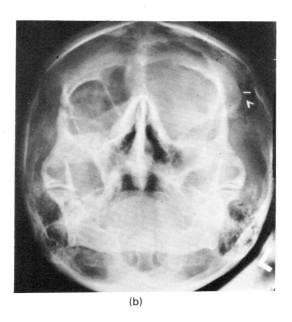
(b)

Fig. 7.2. Left frontal mucocoele. (a) Facial appearance; (b) Radiograph.

REFERENCES

Andrewes C H 1975 In: Viruses in vertebrates. Bailliere Tindall, London, p 23

Dingle J H, Badger G F, Jordan W S Jr 1964 Patterns of illness. In: Illness in the home, Cleveland, Western Reserve University, p 347

Drettner B 1967 International rhinology. Second European congress of rhinology. London, Revue de laryngology, 1 and 2

Drettner B, Lindholm C E 1967 Acta Otolaryngologica Stockholm 64:508

Gwaltney J M Jr, Sydnor A, Sande M A 1981 Etiology and antimicrobial treatment of acute sinusitis. Annals of Otology, Rhinology and Laryngology. 90 (Suppl 84) 3: 68–71

Hope Simpson R E 1958 Symposium on the epidermiology of non-infectious diseases. (a) Common upper respiratory diseases. Royal Society of Health Journal 78:593

Schuknecht, H., Kirmura, R and Naufal P 1973 The pathology of sudden deafiness. Acta Otolaryngologica 76:75

Tyrrell D A J 1981 Prevention of colds. General Practitioner Feb 6:35

Zaiman E, Balducci D, Tyrrell A J 1955 A P C viruses and respiratory disease in Northern England. Lancet ii:595

8
Vasomotor rhinitis

In vasomotor rhinitis disturbances of vascularity in the nose give rise to sneezing, rhinorrhoea and nasal obstruction. The condition underlies most cases of 'nasal catarrh'.

The cause of vasomotor rhinitis may be allergic or non-allergic. Non-allergic rhinitis is often referred to as 'vasomotor rhinitis', but as vasomotor disturbances are common to both groups the former term is less confusing.

ALLERGIC RHINITIS

Allergic rhinitis may be seasonal or perennial. The usual mechanism is a Type 1 immediate hypersensitivity reaction, associated with high IgE levels. A Type III delayed reaction, in which the antigen – antibody complex activates phagocytes leading to vessel wall damage, may less commonly be involved, either accompanying the Type 1 reaction or alone.

Hay fever

The commonest form of allergy in the UK, affecting some 10% of the population, gives rise to symptoms most years from late May until mid-July.

In essence it seems that sufferers differ from 'normal' persons in that they develop large amounts of IgE in response to normal exposure to pollen in the atmosphere. The serum of hay fever sufferers has a mean IgE level two to three times greater than controls (Johansson, 1969). The aetiology of atopy is uncertain. It is sometimes associated in infancy with IgA deficiency and it has been suggested that IgA deficiency at mucosal surfaces permits excessive antigen entry with an over-stimulation of IgE precursors. It has been shown that infants of atopic parents purely breast-fed for the first 6 months are less likely to develop atopy themselves. Avoidance of antigens until maturation of the IgA system, and of ill-understood tolerance – inducing mechanisms, may account for this benefit.

Antigens from pollen grains on the nasal epithelium penetrate the mucosal lining, and are 'processed' by macrophages which stimulate IgE production by T and B lymphocytes. IgE becomes coated on mast cells. On re-exposure, antigen penetrating the mucosa becomes linked to the IgE causing degranulation and breakdown of the mast cells with liberation of various substances including histamine, serotonin, heparin, and chemotoxins.

Clinical picture of hay fever

Exposure to the appropriate pollen results in nasal irritation and itching, recurrent attacks of sneezing, nasal obstruction, and watery rhinorrhoea. The conjunctivae are often affected, with redness, irritation, swollen eyelids and lachrymation. The soft palate is often itchy, and patients may complain of itching ears as a reflex from stimulation of the glossopharyngeal nerve which supplies both areas. Bronchospasm may develop in more severely affected patients. The colour of the nasal mucosa varies widely, from pallor through heliotrope to dull red.

Most hay fever sufferers are allergic to several grass varieties. Italian and perennial rye grasses, and cocksfoot are the most important, being widely grown for hay and silage over Britain. Grass cut for silage is harmless since it is harvested before flowering. Fescue, Yorkshire fog, false oat, and bent grass are also important: they grow in meadows and waste land. Timothy grass pollinates after the main season is over, but is highly allergenic.

Day length determines onset of flowering, and grasses in the South pollinate a week or so earlier than in the Midlands. Cold wet weather in June may delay the onset of the hay fever season, pollen being 'held back' and released in large quantities once fine weather arrives. Conversely hot weather in June may see all the pollen released early, with resulting curtailment of the season.

There is a wide diurnal variation in pollen counts, with low figures at night and early morning, and maximum peaks in the afternoon or evening. In general, symptoms are experienced by most sufferers at above 50 grains/cubic metre, and virtually all are in difficulties at levels above 100 grains/cubic metre. Pollens have been shown to travel 400 miles so that residence in towns gives little protection. Because of widely varying degrees of provocation from day to day and season to season, efficacy of treatment may be difficult to judge.

Diagnosis

The diagnosis of hay fever is plain from the seasonal timing and clinical picture. Routine skin testing against grass pollens adds little.

Management

Whilst complete avoidance of grass pollens during the season is not practicable, patients may be obliged to forego country walks and lawn-mowing during the season.

Antihistamines

These are the mainstay of treatment in hay fever. They inhibit the effects of histamine by blocking H_1 receptors and are effective in relieving sneezing, itching, and rhinorrhoea. Nasal obstruction is less alleviated. The usefulness of antihistamines has been limited by their sedative side effects, resulting from blockage of H_1 receptors in the central nervous system. Recently antihistamines, terfienidine (Priludan) and astemizole (Hismanal), which have been claimed to block peripheral H receptors only have been introduced. Some maintain they have no CNS effects and (unlike older antihistamines) do not potentiate alcohol or diazepam. Astemizole has a very long half-life. Adult doses: terfenadine 60 mg twice daily, astemizole 10 mg daily.

Decongestants

Long-term use of vasoconstrictor nose drops has in the past led through rebound vasodilation to development of rhinitis medicamentosa, in which the nose is severely obstructed by thickened mucosa. Newer decongestants, oxymetazoline (Iliadin – Mini and Afrazine) and xylometazoline (Otrivine) appear not to have this side effect.

Oral decongestants (adrenoceptor stimulants such as ephedrine, pseudoephedrine, phenylephrine and phenylopropanolamine) avoid any risk of damaging the nasal mucosa but more generalised adrenoceptor stimulation restricts their use. They antagonise hypotensive drugs and cause serious reactions in patients receiving monoamine oxidase inhibitors. Pseudoephedrine is marketed alone as Sudafed. Many preparations (Actifed, Benylin Decongestant, Co-Pyronil, Dimotapp, Eskornade, Haymine, Rinurel and Triominic) combine antihistamines with adrenoceptor stimulants. The presence of antihistamine limits day-time use. The long acting Dimotapp LA tablet, one at night, is probably the most successful.

Corticosteroids

Corticosteroids are extremely effective in relieving allergic rhinitis, and can be administered topically, by intramuscular injection, or orally.

a. Beclomethasone (Beconase), betamethasone (Betnesol), budesonide (Rhinocort) and flunisolide (Syntaris) work well: they must be used continuously, twice daily or more. Beclomethasone and budesonide are gaspropelled metered sprays. Betamethasone is supplied as drops, and flunisolide as a metered spray with a pump.

b. Injections of aqueous suspensions of prednisolone (Deltastab), methylprednisolone (Depo-Medrone) and triamcinolone (Kenalog) in a dose of 2 ml are effective in suppressing symptoms of hay fever for at least 2–3 weeks and often for the remainder of the season. They carry the implications of systemic steroid therapy (a blue steroid card should be issued), but are the most helpful treatment for many patients such as candidates sitting higher education examinations.

c. Oral steroids are effective in hay fever, e.g. prednisone 5 mg three times/day reducing to a minimum dose to control symptoms. There is understandable reluctance to prescribe oral steroids for such a common condition as hay fever.

Despite theoretical advantages, ACTH and tetracosactrin (Synacthen) have not established a place in hay fever treatment, their effects being too disseminated and short-lived.

Sodium cromoglycate (SCG)

SCG suppresses both immediate Type 1 allergic reactions and Type 3 delayed reactions. It appears to 'stabilise' the mast cells, preventing them from liberating histamine and other mediators of the allergic response. It is available as a powder, drops (Rynacrom) or spray (Lomusol, Rynacrom).

Whilst SCG is clinically useful, and devoid of any harmful side effects, it has to be introduced into the nose four to six times/day to be effective. Its effect is purely prophylactic, the protection from each dose taking several hours to become effective. It is important to explain this to the patient, otherwise the treatment will be discarded as useless. In practice SCG has proved less important and valuable in allergic rhinitis than in asthma.

Where conjunctival symptoms of hay fever are troublesome, SCG in the form of Opticrom eye drops four times/day is helpful.

Hyposensitising injections

The place for hyposensitising injections in hay fever remains controversial. Some hold them to be ineffective and dangerous (fatal reactions have occurred). Their mode of action is uncertain. It has been postulated that injections of antigen stimulates production of IgG which acts as a 'blocking' antibody. Alternatively, there is evidence that IgE synthesis is suppressed by antigen injections. Others believe tolerance is induced through mechanisms as yet not understood. The allergen – neutralising capacity of post-hyposensitisation serum has been clearly demonstrated (Munro-Ashman et al, 1971). Many physicians and patients are, from experience, convinced of the value of hyposensitising injections. They are better reserved for persons over 12 years of age as before this results are more uncertain and reactions more often severe.

The introduction of tyrosine adsorbed vaccine (Pollinex, containing extracts of pollens from 12 common grasses) has enabled the course of hyposensitising injections to be reduced to three, given at intervals of 1 or 2 weeks.

The course of injections should be completed before onset of the hay fever season. Injections are given subcutaneously, and the syringe plunger should be pulled before injection to ensure the needle is not in a vein. Patients should remain under observation for at least 20 min after injections. For more sensitive patients the risk of adverse reactions may be reduced by administration of an antihistamine 30 min before.

An emergency tray should be kept in readiness wherever desensitising injections are given, containing a supply of needles, syringes, skin swabs and ampoules of Adrenaline 1 in 1000 injection

BP, Aminophylline injection BP, and Hydrocortisone injection BP. In the event of bronchospasm or a more severe generalised reaction the patient should be laid down, 0.5 ml of Adrenaline BP injected subcutaneously at the vaccine injection site, and Aminophylline injection 250–500 mg and if necessary Hydrocortisone 100 mg, both given intravenously. The subcutaneous adrenaline injection may be repeated every 10–15 min if necessary to a total of 2 ml (these doses are for adults).

In the event of bronchospasm or more serious reaction the hyposensitisation course must be abandoned. Courses should be repeated each spring for at least 3 years.

Other forms of seasonal rhinitis

Several trees, pollinating in May and June, give rise to seasonal rhinitis. Spores of moulds and fungi causing allergic rhinitis are prevalent in July and August, and pollens of weeds in August and September.

Symptoms and management are the same as with hay fever, except that identification requires skin testing. A specific vaccine for the allergen or allergens responsible may then be ordered.

Perennial rhinitis

Perennial rhinitis may conveniently be defined as a condition in which at least two of the following symptoms occur for at least an hour on most days:

1. Bouts of sneezing
2. Clear rhinorrhoea
3. Nasal obstruction

In addition there may be nasal irritation, conjunctivitis, reduced sense of smell and taste, and associated sinusitis or nasal polypi. Some patients have a combination of perennial symptoms with seasonal exacerbations. The cause of perennial rhinitis may be either allergic or non-allergic.

1. Allergic perennial rhinitis

The commonest cause of allergic perennial rhinitis in Europe is the house-dust mite *Dermatophagoides pteronyssinus* (*D. Farinae* in North America). Moulds, and food allergy are also important causes. Domestic pets or allergens at work may be responsible.

A careful history must be taken: this often gives a strong clue as to the responsible allergen. It may emerge that symptoms are not severe and that the patient is seeking reassurance rather than active treatment. A family or past history of atopy supports an allergic cause for symptoms. Timing and locality of symptoms are important: housedust mite allergy sufferers often report violent sneezing on making the bed.

Investigation. Anterior rhinoscopy should always be performed, on a day when no treatment has been taken. The nasal mucosa may be of varying shades but is typically moist and swollen. Engorged inferior turbinates sometimes completely obstruct the airway. A local vasoconstrictor (such as cocaine spray or ephedrine 1% drops) should be used if necessary to shrink the mucosa in order to examine the nose for the presence of polypi.

Skin testing. Skin testing helps to confirm allergy suspected from the history. Results must be interpreted with caution as demonstration of hypersensitivity to a particular allergen does not necessarily confirm that this is the cause of the patient's symptoms. Nevertheless, skin testing is the most useful investigation available in allergic rhinitis and is often much appreciated by the patient. It is a simple procedure, suitably performed by a properly instructed practice nurse, and the time needed is less than 30 min. Kits complete with a range of test solutions, stylets, and gauges for measuring skin reaction size are available commercially (e.g. from Bencard), and the cost may be reclaimed from the NHS.

First it must be established that no antihistamines have been taken by the patient during the preceding 48 hours since this would invalidate the tests (steroid therapy however is permissible).

It is convenient to number the test bottles (including the control) then to re-write the numbers in a vertical column on the patient's forearms with a dash opposite each. A small blob from each test bottle is placed on the skin near the end of the corresponding numbered dash using the rod incorporated in each stopper. It is then a simple matter to prick the skin through each blob with the needle supplied in the kit, rinsing and drying it between pricks. The column of blobs can be 'blotted' with a paper towel (taking care to avoid cross contaminating the test sites) and the patient is left for 15–20 min. The results are then read, measuring the diameter of any reactions (Fig. 8.1).

RAST (Radioallergosorbent test) is a sensitive method for measuring IgE to particular antigens *in vitro*. Most district hospital laboratories can now screen blood for raised IgE levels to specific

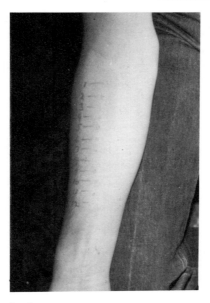

Fig. 8.1 Skin testing in progress.

allergens: over 150 different allergens are covered. These tests, and total IgE level measurements, can be performed on a 3 ml sample of blood. The results of RAST tests correlate well with skin tests. RAST tests give quantifiable results but tell little more than skin tests, which are so much quicker and cheaper to perform.

Food allergy

The importance and frequent occurrence of food allergy has been increasingly appreciated in recent years. Cows milk protein, eggs, wheat, fermented drinks, colouring agents including tartrazines and citrus fruits are amongst ingested allergens most commonly responsible for perennial rhinitis. Skin tests are of no value in detecting many cases of food allergy. In theory RAST tests should be more dependable, quantifying specific IgE to suspected food allergens. In practice, however, too many false positive and false negatives are obtained for the method to be useful.

At present only one reliable way of identifying allergens in the diet is available, by successive exclusion of dietary components for a period of up to 1 month. When relief of symptoms occurs following elimination of a particular foodstuff, its suspected complicity can be challenged by reintroducing it to the diet. General practitioners may find the help of the district hospital dietician invaluable in investigating patients for food allergens, and constructing nutritionally adequate diets to be followed subsequently, where a food allergen is identified.

Management of allergic perennial rhinitis

Management involves avoidance of identified allergens, and antiallergic measures as used in seasonal rhinitis. For hyposensitisation to the housedust mite a specific vaccine (Migen Bencard) is available. An initial course of six injections at 1–2-week intervals is followed by long-term monthly maintenance doses.

Chronic hypertrophic rhinitis

This may develop in longstanding cases of either allergic or non-allergic perennial rhinitis. Poor shrinkage of the turbinates on application of vasoconstrictor drops indicates the presence of fibrosis. A large pale 'mulberry-like' swelling of the posterior ends of the inferior turbinates may be visible on posterior rhinoscopy, and may be the cause of considerable nasal obstruction. Surgical resection may be required.

2. Non-allergic perennial rhinitis

Perennial rhinitis can only be classified as non-allergic if no evidence of allergy can be found on skin testing, and if necessary, dietary exclusion investigations. The dividing line between allergic and non-allergic rhinitis is not sharp: in many cases an allergic cause is strongly suspected but cannot be confirmed by techniques so far available.

The turbinates are capable of great variation in size and wetness in order to fulfil their role in warming, humidifying, and filtering inspired air. The capacity to vary so much in size is provided by richly innervated cavernous erectile tissue.

Fenestration of the epithelial layer of capillaries in the turbinate mucosa and porosity of the overlying ciliated mucous membrane assists in the moisturising function.

The erectile tissue and mucous glands are under autonomic control. Sympathetic stimulation leads to shrinkage of the turbinates and paleness and dryness of the mucosa; parasympathetic stimulation causes swelling of the turbinates with hyperaemia and hypersecretion. It is thought that the hypothalamus regulates the autonomic outflow to the nasal mucosa, co-ordinating impulses, including emotional stimuli, from higher centres. Circulating hormones and some drugs have a direct effect on the mucosa, as do changes in atmospheric temperature and humidity. Fright causes a sympathetic reaction, with vasoconstriction, whilst anxiety typically leads to a parasympathetic reaction with nasal obstruction and hypersecretion.

In health, the nasal airway is alternately widened on one side then the other, each cycle lasting from 5 min to several hours. This fluctuation is not noticed in health but may lead to troublesome intermittent obstruction if the airway is already impaired.

Causative factors in non-allergic rhinitis

Emotional factors. These are most important, stress and anxiety leading to autonomic overstimulation. The much greater incidence in a suburban population where 'rat race' problems are common as compared with a provincial semi-rural practice is striking. Emotional factors are also at work in 'honeymoon rhinitis'.

Drugs. Antihypertensive drugs such as a adrenergic blocking agents, including guanethidine (Ismelin), and catecholamine–depleting agents such as reserpine and methyldopa (Aldomet) may cause nasal stuffiness. Ergot preparations have sympathetic blocking effects and may also cause nasal stuffiness. Drugs with anticholinesterase action may too cause nasal obstruction by potentiating acetylcholine.

Environmental factors. In many non-allergic rhinitis sufferers, the fault appears to lie in exaggeration of normal responsiveness of the nasal mucosa to cold, dust particles in the air, and changing humidity.

Clinical picture

In some patients the principal complaint is of nasal obstruction; in others it is excessive rhinorrhoea. In others, both symptoms are equally troublesome, and there may be frequent bouts of sneezing. Women of childbearing age with non-allergic rhinitis are particularly susceptible to excessive rhinorrhoea. They are sometimes psychologically unstable and resistant to treatment.

Management

Reassurance, and the knowledge that their symptoms are understood and that genuine efforts are being made to help them, is of great importance to patients. Allergy must have been excluded.

Somewhat paradoxically antihistamines are often helpful in non-allergic rhinitis and are conveniently given in combination with a-stimulators as Dimotapp LA tablets, one at night.

By its anticholinergic side effect imipramine 25–50 mg at night often reduces severe rhinorrhoea.

Intranasal topical steroids such as beclomethasone (Beconase) are helpful: the full benefit may not be apparent until 1 month's use.

All practicable steps should be taken to reduce stress where this appears to be implicated.

Surgery

Medical management should always be given a thorough trial. For very resistant cases surgery may be needed. Submucosal diathermy is simple and often effective in reducing turbinate enlargement. Surgical reduction of the turbinates and lateral fracture of the inferior turbinates is often helpful but subject to the reservation that the nasal anatomy can thereafter never return to normal.

There is a strong tendency for adhesions to form between the septum and the turbinates after such operations. These can be largely avoided by leaving a sheet of silastic (a 'nasal splint') in each nasal cavity, held in place by a stitch transfixing both splints and the front of the nasal septum, after operation. The splints are removed 2 weeks later in the out-patient department after dividing the suture.

For patients with excessive watery rhinorrhoea, resistant to treatment, and who are emotionally stable, the operation of division of the nerve of the pterygoid canal (Vidian neurectomy) may give relief. The procedure is technically difficult and should only be undertaken by surgeons with practice.

Surgery for perennial rhinitis is only indicated in a small proportion of resistant cases, and the great majority are best cared for in general practice.

REFERENCES

Johansson S G O 1969 Proceedings of the Royal Society of Medicine 62:975
Munro-Ashman D, McEwen H, Feinberg J G 1971 The patient-self (PS) test. Demonstration of a rise in blocking antibodies after treatment with Allpyrol. International Archives of Allergy and Applied Immunology 40:448

9

Nasal polypi

Nature

Nasal polypi are essentially pieces of oedematous upper respiratory mucosa attached to their site of origin by a stalk. They can arise from any part of the nasal or sinus mucosa. Most arise from the middle and anterior ethmoid groups of air cells and protrude into the middle meatus. Some arise from the posterior ethmoid group and lie in the superior meatus beneath the superior turbinate. Some arise and remain in other sinuses. One particular type, the antro-choanal polyp, arises in the maxillary antrum, enters the nose through the ostium, and passes backwards on the floor of the nasal cavity to enter the post-nasal space through the posterior choana.

Ninety per cent of nasal polypi are infiltrated with eosinophils and excess eosinophils can also be demonstrated in nasal smears. They are sometimes associated with non-allergic asthma and with aspirin intolerance. 10 per cent of nasal polypi in adults are infiltrated with neutrophils. They are often associated with infected sinuses and purulent nasal discharge. In children neutrophil polypi may be associated with cystic fibrosis, and their presence calls for a sweat test.

Causes of nasal polypi

Polypi develop as a result of accumulation of intercellular fluid due either to local vascular disturbance or to the Bernouilli phenomenon, negative pressure developing close to the site of restricted airflow and encouraging tissue oedema. Allergic processes and infections may both be involved in the formation of polypi, acting singly or together.

Clinical picture

Small polypi may cause no symptoms. Medium sized polypi often cause intermittent obstruction, sometimes with a 'valve' effect, breathing in being easier than breathing out. Larger polypi cause complete obstruction, and, if bilateral, continual mouth breathing. Complete obstruction is often precipitated by onset of a cold. Anosmia is usual.

Recognition

The presence of nasal polypi is usually obvious on anterior rhinoscopy. Where the turbinate mucosa is thickened it may be necessary to spray the nose with a decongestant to obtain a satisfactory view. A cocaine or xylocaine spray is particularly useful, enabling use of a probe in the nose to determine whether tissue resembling polypi is mobile on a stalk.

Antro-choanal polypi are sometimes large enough to be visible through the mouth – hanging down into the pharynx from behind the soft palate. Otherwise they may only be visible on posterior rhinoscopy.

Management

Apart from causing nasal obstruction polypi interfere with the mucociliary system and predispose to infection. Treatment is therefore usually called for. Surgical removal of polypi will usually be required, and this can often be performed satisfactorily in adults under local anaesthesia in the ENT out-patient department. For children, or where numerous polypi are present, a much more satisfactory clearance can be performed under general anaesthesia.

Steroid treatment, either systemic or intranasally (as beclomethasone 'Beconase') often results in considerable shrinkage or even disappearance of the common eosinophilic type of polypi.

When nasal polyi are encountered in general practice, referral to an ENT department is usually called for. Where there is long delay in appointments, and particularly if sinus disease is excluded radiologically, considerable relief may be provided by prescription of a beclomethasone (Beconase) spray, two puffs to be directed into each nostril at varying directions in the sagittal plane, two or three times/day.

10

Epistaxis

Epistaxis is probably the commonest type of haemorrhage the general practitioner is called upon to treat.

Little's area

Bleeding usually comes from Little's area, a point on the anterior inferior part of the septum where the ethmoidal, greater palatine, sphenoplatine and superior labial arteries anastomose. In this region some of the vessels may be poorly supported and the overlying epithelium frail. In young people, a vein running vertically at the anterior edge of Little's area on its way to the floor of the nose is vulnerable. Blowing the nose, breathing excessively dry air, physical activity, minor trauma, and upper respiratory infection, or raised blood pressure may then be sufficient to precipitate bleeding. Very often the immediate cause of bleeding is a mystery.

Bleeding from further back in the nose is much less common, and is seen chiefly in elderly arteriosclerotic patients. Very serious bleeding occurs from the nasopharynx in juvenile angiofibroma, a condition affecting males between the ages of 10 and 20 years, which though rare, should be borne in mind particularly by doctors responsible for youngsters at school or in the Forces.

Anticoagulant therapy, and blood disorders such as thrombocytopaenic purpura, leukaemia and sickle cell anaemia predispose to epistaxes.

A rare though important cause is hereditary telangiectasia (Osler's disease) transmitted as a Mendelian dominant. There is often no evidence of this disease until adult life, when aggregations of minute vessels begin to appear scattered over the mucous membrane of the nose, mouth, pharynx, and skin of the face, neck and arms. The patients usually present with epistaxes and the multiple lesions are noted.

Management of epistaxis

By the time medical help is requested, a patient with an epistaxis, and his relatives, have often become somewhat excited. A physiologically insignificant volume of blood, distributed amongst numerous tissues and old rags, may appear to them to constitute a dangerous haemorrhage. The general alarm may elevate the patient's blood pressure, aggravating the bleeding. The doctor's first task therefore is to introduce an atmosphere of calm and reassurance. The patient should be advised to sit upright, with his head tilted slightly forwards, so that he can drip and spit into a bowl, and the nose should be firmly pinched between thumb and fingers for 5–10 min. He should breathe through his mouth. As most bleeding is from Little's area, and this will be compressed when the nose is pinched, on releasing pressure the bleeding will usually have stopped. The patient's blood pressure should be recorded and if elevated, hypotensive treatment may be begun at once.

When compression is released, the nose may be gently inspected, using a Thudichum's speculum, to locate the bleeding point. If this can be identified, and the bleeding recurs, it can be cauterised later. If, on the other hand, no bleeding point can be seen, and bleeding continues, it must be coming from further back. This is most common in arteriosclerotic patients, and hospital admission is often advisable. However an attempt should be made to compress the unseen bleeding point and this may be done either by packing the nose with gauze tape, or with an inflatable bag such as Simpson's or Brighton's inflatable tampon.

Unanointed gauze is traumatic to nasal mucosa, and encourages putrefaction. Gauze is traditionally impregnated with BIPP (bismouth iodoform paraffin paste), available in tubes (Fig. 10.1). Some of the paste is squeezed into a bowl and a length of tape immersed in it before use. Failing this, the gauze can be lubricated with paraffin. Simpson's and Brighton's tampons are effective but usually seem to be unavailable or perished.

Whichever method is used, the nose should be sprayed with 10% cocaine solution unless the rate of bleeding makes this useless.

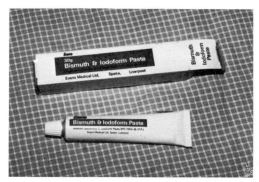

Fig. 10.1. Bismuth and Iodoform paste available in tube form.

Tape packings are built up in layers inside the nose from below upwards. If a Simpson's tampon is used, after introduction 6–10 ml of air is injected with a disposable syringe and it is taped in position with strapping.

A pair of angled forceps (e.g. Pritchard's), a Thudichum's speculum, and good illumination are needed.

If, despite such packing, bleeding continues, hospital admission is indicated, where introduction of a pack or balloon into the post nasal space may be required, and of course blood transfusion may be necessary. Death from coronary thrombosis secondary to hypotension resulting from epistaxis appears regularly in the

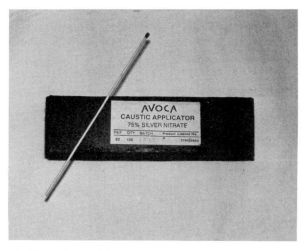

Fig. 10.2. Silver nitrate sticks.

168   EAR, NOSE AND THROAT DISORDERS

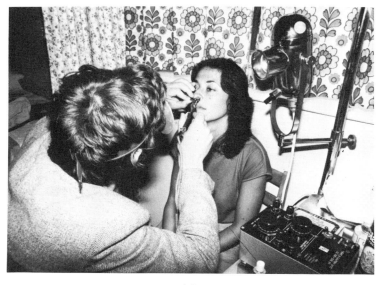

(a)

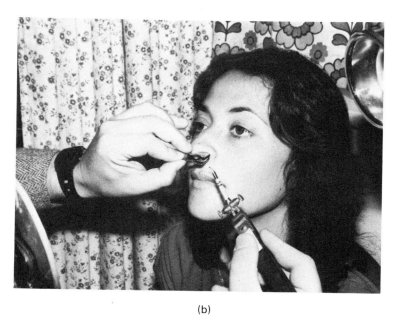

(b)

Fig. 10.3. (a) and (b) Electrocautery set in use.

Registrar-General's mortality statistics. On rare occasions arterial ligation proves necessary (ligation of the anterior ethmoid on the medial wall of the orbit or branches of the external carotid artery, depending on whether bleeding is from above or below the middle turbinate).

Cauterisation

If a persistently or recurrently bleeding site can be visualised, it may be cauterised after local anaesthesia with 10% cocaine spray or a Xylocaine spray. Caustics such as silver nitrate [ready-made silver nitrate sticks (Fig. 10.2) are convenient], chromium trioxide or trichloracetic acid (applied on the end of a cotton wool pleget mounted on a Jobson Horne probe) may be used. Care must be taken that application of caustic is confined to the bleeding area. Alternatively, electrocautery may be used: it provides more dependable coagulation and is readily available in many general practices nowadays (Fig. 10.3). A short electrode should be used – electrodes several inches long designed for cautery of the cervix are too unweildy.

Epistaxis in hereditary telangectasia presents a special problem: it is often difficult to determine which of the multiple lesions is the source of bleeding on any one occasion. These patients should be referred for hospital care: repeated blood transfusions are often required. Oestrogens have been claimed to be helpful, and skin grafting inside the nose has been employed.

Treatment of epistaxis in the patient's home, with makeshift facilities and inadequate lighting, is seldom satisfactory. The properly equipped general practitioner can deal with the great majority of epistaxes in his surgery. Bleeding in older patients, not controlled by pinching, is likely to be coming from further back in the nose and hospital care will generally be needed.

11

Injuries to the nose and snoring

INJURIES TO THE NOSE

Two types of injury are common – lateral displacements arising from a sideward blow, and broadening of the nasal bridge produced by a frontal blow. Septal injuries may accompany either type.

It is sometimes difficult to appreciate the degree of deformity when face to face with the patient. A better assessment is obtained by standing behind the seated patient whose head is tilted backwards. The examiner looks down at the patient's nose with the forehead as a 'foreground'. Any deformity then becomes more obvious.

If the patient is seen immediately after injury, and he has a lateral displacement, the fragments are usually quite mobile. It may be possible, as a 'first aid' measure, to push the nose straight by pressure with the thumb against the displaced side of the nasal bones. More usually, manipulation under anaesthesia will be required, and the patient should be seen in a casualty department as soon as possible. If several hours have passed since the injury, there is likely to be so much swelling that accurate correction of the deformity will not be possible. This swelling usually takes about 6 days to subside, and thereafter the displaced bones will remain easily manipulable for a further 2 weeks or so. Later than this, correction of the deformity will be a more difficult procedure, involving refracture of the nasal bones.

Radiography is not of great help in the management of nasal injuries: it gives little more information than clinical examination.

SNORING

Patients occasionally present is general practice considerably distressed by snoring. Much animosity may be engendered within a household, and marriages may be jeopardised. Severe snoring is sometimes associated with sleep apnoea in adults. The source of most loud snoring is the soft palate, which partially obstructs the airway during sleep.

Hitherto no dependable remedy has been available, but a highly promising operation has now been described 'uvulopalatopharyngoplasty' (Simmons et al, 1983). The procedure involves excision of the uvula, and a rim of soft palate and anterior faucial pillar (Fig. 11.).

Of a series of eight patients who underwent uvulopalatopharyngoplasty for socially unacceptable snoring, all were cured. The theoretically possible complications of palatal stenosis, troublesome lasting nasal regurgitation, or 'nasal' speech, did not occur.

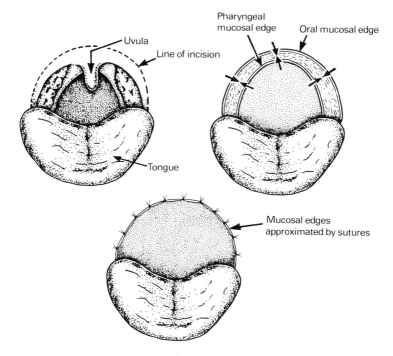

Fig. 11.1. Uvulopalatopharyngoplasty.

The suggested criteria for consideration of the operation are:

1. snoring loud enough to be heard at least one room away or where the bed partner has moved elsewhere, and

2. snoring should be independant of sleeping position on side, back, or stomach.

REFERENCE

Simmons F B, Guilleminault C, Silverstri R 1983 Snoring, and some obstructive sleep apnoea, can be cured by oropharyngeal surgery. Palatopharyngoplasty. Archives of Otolaryngology 109: 503–507

Part 4
The Pharynx and Larynx

12

Anatomy and examination of the pharynx and the larynx

The pharynx

The pharynx extends from the base of the skull to the beginning of the oesophagus, and is divided into the nasopharynx above the soft palate, the oropharynx between soft palate and base of tongue, and the laryngopharynx below. Fig. 12.1.

Waldeyer's ring

Composed of lymphoid tissue this forms a band around the upper respiratory and digestive tracts (Fig. 12.2). The main components are the adenoids and faucial tonsils. The lingual tonsils, pharyngeal lymph nodes, and lymphoid aggregations above and behind the openings of the Eustachian tubes in the nasopharynx complete the ring.

The adenoids

These are situated on the posterior wall of the nasopharynx and are thrown into a series of longitudinal ridges enlarging their surface area. The tissue immediately beneath the surface epithelium is lymphoid, and arranged in nodules, some with germ centres. Loose lymphatic tissue separates the nodules. The surface epithelium is infiltrated with lymphocytes.

The faucial tonsils

These lie in a triangular fossa formed by the palatoglossal and palatopharyngeal folds and the base of the tongue (Fig. 12.3). The

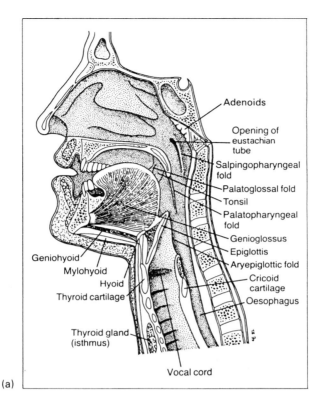

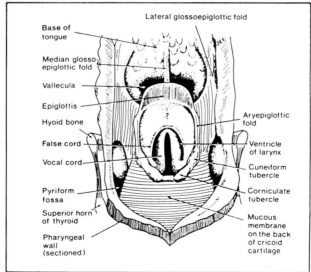

Fig. 12.1. (a) Sagittal section through nasal cavity, pharynx and larynx.
(b) Anatomical diagram of anterior wall of laryngo-pharynx viewed from behind.

EXAMINATION OF PHARYNX   177

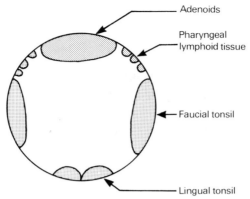

Fig. 12.2. Waldeyer's ring.

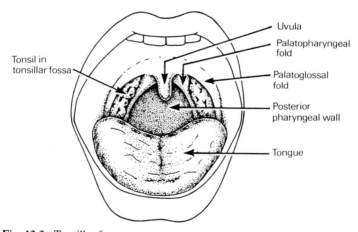

Fig. 12.3. Tonsillar fossa

palatoglossal fold may largely conceal the tonsil, but during contraction of the superior constrictor muscles during swallowing the tonsils are 'extruded' into the pharynx. Between 10 and 30 crypts descend from the surface of the tonsil, penetrating almost to its base. Epithelium lined extensions project from them, greatly increasing the surface epithelial area. Sub-epithelial lymphoid tissue is thus brought into contact with the environment of the oral and pharyngeal cavities. As well as organisms, the crypts contain desquamated cells and debris. Lymphocytes from the lymphoid tissue escape into the mouth. Although mucous glands are present, their ducts do not open into the bases of the crypts, so that stagnation and infection at the bottom of the crypts is prone to occur.

The lingual tonsil

This is a collection of lymphatic tissue at the root of the tongue resembling the faucial tonsil in general and microscopic structure but possessing mucous glands with ducts opening at the crypt bases. The resulting flushing action has been held responsible for the freedom of the lingual tonsil from disease.

Lymphoid nodules are inconspicuous in health but may become prominant, particularly in the presence of viral infection.

Role of lymphoid tissue in Waldeyer's Ring

Functions of lymphoid tissue generally include the following.

1. Formation of lymphocytes.
2. Removal of micro-organisms, bacterial toxins, extravascular proteins and foreign particles from lymph.
3. Cellular defence against infection. Plasma cells and small round cells, fibroblasts and macrophages are derived from lymphocytes or their precursors. Lymphocytes themselves probably play only a small phagocytic role, but provide proteolytic enzymes, and are a source of antibodies.
4. Antibody synthesis. This occurs in the plasma cells, differentiated from lymphocytes during antibody synthesis.
5. Lymphoid tissue incorporates reticulo-endothelial elements whose function is active phagocytosis.

The pharyngeal lymphoid tissues are brought into intimate contact with all that is inhaled and ingested by virtue of their sub-epithelial situation.

It seems that they collect micro-organisms from the nasal passages and mouth, manufacture antibodies, and absorb and modify their toxins, releasing them to the reticulo-endothelial system throughout the body where they stimulate major antibody production. The principal growth of pharyngeal lymphoid tissues occurs in the early years of life, and after the age of 10 years the tissues regress. Presumably this growth pattern reflects the heightened antibody production called for in early years as increasing numbers of antigens are first encountered.

To what extent antibody formation is jeopardised by adenotonsillectomy is still uncertain. There is a strong tendency for remaining elements of Waldeyer's ring to hypertrophy when a portion is extirpated. It is a familiar observation that tonsils often enlarge considerably after adenoidectomy alone has been performed.

Many clinicians are unhappy about the immunological implications of adenotonsillectomy.

The larynx

The larynx is composed of articulated cartilages, with interconnecting ligaments and muscles. It lies opposite the 3rd–6th cervical vertebrae in adult men, and a little higher in women and children. Intrinsic muscles move one cartilage upon another and extrinsic muscles connect the larynx to the surrounding structures.

Of the cartilages three are unpaired: the epiglottis, thyroid, and cricoid cartilages and six are paired: the arytenoids, cuneiform and corniculate cartilages (Fig. 12.4).

The thyroid and cricoid cartilages

The thyroid cartilage is the largest and resembles an open book, the 'back' turned forwards in the midline. The cricoid cartilage lies below and articulates with it. It is shaped somewhat like a signet

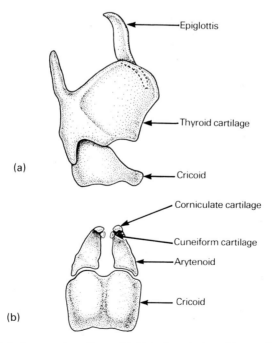

Fig. 12.4. Laryngeal cartilages. (a) Right lateral view. (b) seen from behind.

ring with the 'signet' facing posteriorly and bearing articular facets on either side for articulation with the inferior horn of the thyroid cartilage. Higher up are facets for articulation with the arytenoid cartilage. The 'signet' (or posterior lamina) forms most of the posterior wall of the larynx.

The lower border of the cricoid cartilage is connected to the first ring of the trachea by the cricotracheal ligament.

The paired aryteroid cartilages

These sit on top of the upper and lateral borders of the cricoid posteriorly. Shaped like irregular three-sided pyramids, their medial surfaces are submucus. Each bears two processes: lateral, for attachment of muscle, and anterior (the vocal process) to which the vocal ligaments are attached,

(The two very small paired cuneiform and corniculate cartilages lie within the ary-epiglottic folds.)

The epiglottis

This is a flattened leaf of fibrocartilage attached by its 'stalk' to the top of the thyroid cartilage in the midline.

The free upper border projects upwards and backwards behind the tongue. Folds of mucous membrane (the ary-epiglottic folds) run backwards from the edges from the epiglottis to the arytenoids, and with them form the margins of the entrance to the glottis.

Intrinsic muscles

One group opens and closes the glottis (the aperture between the vocal cords), another controls the tension of the cords, and a third group controls the opening to the larynx.

All but the cricothyroid (which controls tension of the vocal cords), are supplied by the recurrent laryngeal nerve (derived from the vagus). The cricothyroid is innervated by the external branch of the superior laryngeal nerve, also a branch of the vagus.

The cavity of the larynx

This is divided into a superior vestibule lying above the folds of mucosa overlying intrinsic ligaments, (the vestibular folds or 'false cords'), the laryngeal ventricle between 'false' and 'true' cords, and

EXAMINATION OF PHARYNX

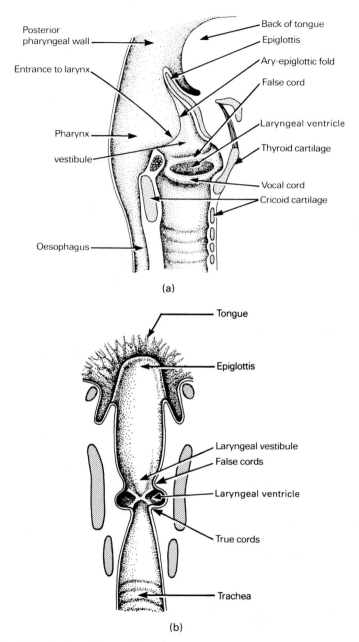

Fig. 12.5. Cavity of larynx (a) lateral. (b) Antero-posterior.

the subglottic region below the true cords (Fig. 12.5). The narrowest part of the upper respiratory tract is in the lower part of the subglottic region, at the level of the cricoid, and it is here that inhaled foreign bodies are likely to be arrested and trauma from endotracheal tubes to occur.

EXAMINATION OF THE PHARYNX AND LARYNX

The oropharynx is under fairly constant scrutiny in general practice, principally in a search for evidence of upper respiratory infection. Smoking habits should always be ascertained: smokers have inflamed pharyngeal mucosa whether or not infection is present.

In younger children dubious of allowing inspection of their throats, the most rewarding approach may be to ask the mother to lay the patient backwards across her knees (Fig. 12.6). Looking at him from the side, 'upside down', it is usually possible to depress the tongue and inspect the throat with little resistance.

Examination of the post nasal space is considered on page 136.

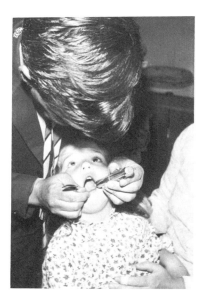

Fig. 12.6. Examination of child's throat.

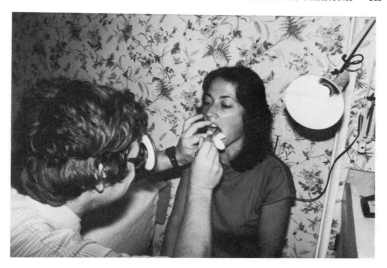

Fig. 12.7. Indirect laryngoscopy.

Indirect laryngoscopy

The larynx is examined using a head mirror or focusing head lamp and a laryngeal mirror. The examiner sits facing the patient who is asked to remove any dentures, sit well back in the chair, tilt his body slightly forwards, open his mouth wide, stick out his tongue, and breathe quietly through his mouth (Fig. 12.7). A laryngeal mirror (the largest convenient) is warmed in a flame and the back touched on the back of the examiner's hand to check it is not too hot. The examiner wraps a gauze swab over the end of the tongue, grips the tongue gently between thumb and finger tips, and draws it forwards.

The light beam is focused on the uvula. The mirror (held like a pencil) is introduced into the mouth with the back resting against the uvula and adjoining soft palate. Great care must be taken that the mirror does not touch the fauces, back of tongue, or posterior pharangeal wall, or the gag reflex will be stimulated. Extreme gentleness is essential. Some patients cannot tolerate the mirror without the help of a local anaesthetic such as a benzocaine lozenge, or a spray with 5% cocaine or Xylocaine.

Manipulating the mirror, the oropharynx, laryngopharynx, and larynx are examined (Fig. 12.8). The pink false cords, and beyond

184 EAR, NOSE AND THROAT DISORDERS

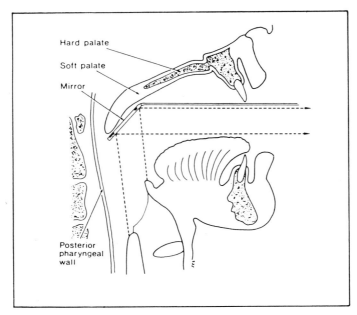

Fig. 12.8. Indirect laryngoscopy. Anterior structures are seen at the 'top' of the mirror, posterior structures at the 'bottom'.

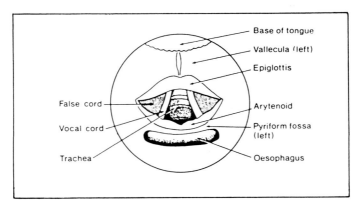

Fig. 12.9. Diagram of structures as seen in the mirror on indirect laryngoscopy.

them the pale vocal cords are inspected, and their mobility on inspiration and phonation (the patient is asked to say 'haaay') ascertained. It is often possible to see well down the trachea (Fig. 12.9).

Patients vary considerably in the ease with which their larynges may be examined. Much depends on rapport, and the examiner's success in getting them to relax and co-operate. Some patients start to 'gag' as soon as the mirror approaches their mouth, and satisfactory examination may be impossible in even the most experienced hands. Physical problems may also defeat the examination, as in cervical spondylosis or 'infantile' configuration of the epiglottis.

13
Tonsil and adenoid problems

ACUTE TONSILLITIS

Aetiology

Adenoviruses are the commonest groups of viruses involved in tonsillitis. Bacterial infection may be secondary to viral invasion, or may occur 'de novo' in debilitated patients, where the tonsils are diseased from previous infections, or where the bacteria concerned are of particular virulence.

The commonest bacterium encountered in tonsillitis is the haemolytic streptococcus. In an on-going study within sentinel practices in the Oxford region, group A streptococci were isolated from 17% of sore throats, and group B, C and G streptococci from another 3.7%. Other pathogens (*Haemophilus influenzae* and *Staphylococcus aureus*) were isolated from 1.2% of sore throats. Virus culture and serological techniques identified adenoviruses, Coxsackie, rhinoviruses and para-influenza viruses in a further 10–20%. (Figures reported from Epidemiological Research Unit, Guildford.) Caution must however be exercised in interpreting the significance of throat swabs. Many bacteria can adopt either a commensal or a pathogenic role, and it is often uncertain whether a cultured organism is truely causal. Recent interest has focused on the aetiological importance of anaerobic organisms in tonsillitis.

Clinical appearance

Three forms of tonsillitis are described.

1. Acute follicular tonsillitis: whitish or yellowish spots of purulent exudate mark the reddened surface: this is the commonest picture in haemolytic streptococcal infection.

2. Acute parenchymatous tonsillitis, where the whole tonsil is swollen and red.

3. Acute membranous tonsillitis, where exudate from crypts has coalesced to form a confluent membrane.

These appearances usually merely represent different stages of the same disease process.

Microscopically inflammation of the tonsil is accompanied by hyperaemia and oedema, and conversion of lymphoid follicles into abscesses which discharge into the crypts.

Age incidence

The peak incidence of tonsillitis is in the fifth and sixth years (Fig. 13.1), with a further low wide peak in teenagers and young adults suffering from infectious mononucleosis. Tonsillitis is rare in infancy and after the age of 50 years.

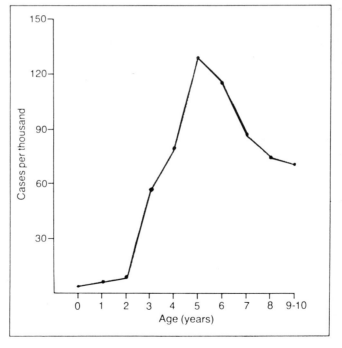

Fig. 13.1. Annual prevalence of acute tonsilitis in children. Courtesy of Dr J. Fry.

Diagnosis

Although children with tonsillitis may complain of a sore throat, general malaise and fever are more frequent presenting symptoms, and throat infections are the commonest cause of abdominal pain in children. A characteristic foetid smell in the breath is often noticeable.

On inspecting the throat the diagnosis is usually obvious at a glance.

In older patients with small infected tonsils, care must be taken to look deep into the tonsillar fossa, or the diagnosis may be missed.

The jugulo-digastic and posterior triangle lymph nodes should instinctively be palpated: enlargement of the latter accompanies adenoidal infection.

Differential diagnosis

Appearances clinically indistinguishable from other types of tonsillitis occur in infectious mononucleosis. This is to be suspected in young adults developing persistent and recurring sore throats after a 2–3-week period of vague ill health. Enlargement of lymph nodes other than those in the neck, and splenomegaly, should be looked for, and blood examined for Paul Bunnell and differential white cell count.

Vincent's angina

This is a subacute tonsillitis with ulceration, sometimes unilateral, and is rare in children. Exudate leads to membrane and slough formation which on separating leaves an irregular excavating ulcer. Foetor is marked. Associated Vincent's fusiform bacilli and *Spirochaeta denticolata* are the causative organisms and may be cultered from a throat swab.

Scarlatina

Scarlatina consists of tonsillitis or pharyngitis due to Lancefield's group A streptococci, associated with general effects arising from soluble toxins, one of which causes a punctate erythematous rash in susceptible patients. There is likely to be stippling of the palate, a 'strawberry' tongue, fever and pronounced tachycardia. Confirmation is by throat swab. Nephritis is common after infection with

Griffith's type 12, 4, and 25 streptococci. Rheumatic fever and carditis have been reported associated with type M5.

Diphtheria

Diphtheria typically causes membrane formation, eventually greenish black, over the tonsil. The membrane may spread onto the faucial pillars and soft palate and removal causes bleeding. Marked lymph gland enlargement is usually present. Identification of the Klebs–Löffler bacillus by swab of the membrane is diagnostic, but treatment with antiserum and penicillin should be begun without awaiting bacteriological reports if diagnosis seems likely on clinical grounds. If antitoxin is delayed more than 72 hours after the development of symptoms it will have little effect on morbidity or mortality. Harmless diphtheroids cannot be distinguished from *Corynebacterium diphtheriae* by light microscopy and Gram staining, and confirmation has to await culture.

Although diphtheria has been almost eradicated in Brirain as a result of widespread immunisation, notoriety mistakenly attached to pertussis immunisation has resulted in a general decline in take-up of all forms of immunisation. A rise in numbers of persons susceptible to diphtheria can be anticipated, and the risk is increased by arrival in the UK of unimmunised visitors from underdeveloped countries where the disease is still a major killer. The general practitioner's alertness to the possible significance of an adherant membrane in the throat of a toxic patient is crucial.

Blood dyscrasias and leukaemia may be associated with throat infections as a consequence of breakdown of immunological defences. Ulceration and bleeding in gums and elswhere in the pharynx raise suspicion, and call for blood examination.

Management

Indications for antibiotics

Although indiscriminate administration of antibiotics is deplored, certain considerations support the prescription of antibiotics for patients with acute tonsillitis.

1. Uncontrolled bacterial infection is likely to cause permanent damage to tonsillar architecture, with chronic infection, micro-abscess formation, and fibrosis. Timely antibiotic administration should avoid this morbidity.

2. No visual criteria exists enabling differentiation between viral and bacterial tonsillitis. Nor are throat swabs of much help in making this distinction, for organisms isolated and held responsible for tonsillitis are also encountered in healthy persons, and pathogenic organisms (including anaerobic bacteria) may be concealed in tonsil crypts and absent from throat swabs. All infected tonsils must therefore be considered potential harbourers of bacterial infection, amenable to antibiotic therapy.

3. The considerable decline in incidence of acute glomerulonephritis and of rheumatic fever in the last three to four decades remains unexplained. Some would credit decreased virulence of haemolytic streptococci, and improved living standards, for this benefit. However antibiotics have been widely used for throat infections during this period and could equally well claim credit (Editorial, The Practitioner, 1983).

4. Man's immunological mechanisms evolved to meet the requirements of small groups living in relative isolation, Circumstances in modern civilisations, with thousands living in close proximity, and children crowded together for education results in early heavy exposure to a wide range of organisms. Judicious use of antibiotics to mitigate some of the difficulties imposed by this highly artificial environment would appear not unreasonable.

In the absence of any degree of certainty as to the cause of tonsillitis in any individual case, scientific management is difficult to plan. Most doctors regard the presence of purulent exudate on the surface of an inflamed tonsil as an indication that bacterial infection is present and that antibiotic treatment is indicated. Others prescribe antibiotics in the presence of tonsillitis with fever whatever the appearances. Yet others take additional factors into account such as the following.

    a. Previous medical history.
    b. Previous response to antibiotics.
    c. General health.
    d. Anticipated likelihood of complications.
    e. Credence given to proposition that antibiotics help prevent chronic tonsil infection.
    f. Patient's and parents' expectations.
    g. Domestic and social circumstances.
    h. Forthcoming programme, e.g. school examinations or imminent holiday.

If antibiotic treatment is to be given, penicillin V is active for most infections (erythromycin in the case of patients allergic to penicillin). Throat swabs (the limitations of their relevance accepted) may guide subsequent antibiotic therapy.

Little benefit can be anticipated from antibiotic administration in tonsillitis accompanying infective mononucleosis, and of course ampicillin and amoxicillin must be avoided in view of the common resultant skin eruption.

Most patients with tonsillitis feel ill and are glad to go to bed. Adult cases often appear to be more toxic and distressed than children. Soluble aspirin (dissolved in water, gargled then swallowed) helps to relieve the sore throat.

Complications of acute tonsillitis

Chronic tonsillitis

This results when recurrent attacks of acute tonsillitis fail to resolve. Abscesses in lymphoid follicles surrounding the tonsillar crypts have become 'walled off' by fibrous tissue and are thus largely inaccessible to antibiotics or to natural immunity processes. Chronically infected tonsils harbour large numbers of organisms: more than 10^5/gram of tissue. These are mostly non-pathogenic, α-streptococci and *Neisseria* predominating (Brook et al, 1980). They are generally associated with complaints of sore throat with fever and malaise more than seven times/year (Saski & Koss, 1978). Adenoids behave similarly (Kyetmetal, 1982).

Group A beta-haemolytic streptococci are present in a minority of chronically infected tonsils, and are isolated twice as often from the tonsil core after tonsillectomy than from the tonsil surface. Many of the aerobic and anaerobic organisms isolated from tonsils removed following recurrent tonsillitis are beta-lactamase producers, capable of preventing penicillin from eradication group A beta-haemolytic streptococci. Alternative antibiotics such as lincomycin, clindamycin or cloxacillin may be preferable to penicillin since they are effective against beta-lactamase producing organisms as well as against streptococci.

Quinsy (peritonsillar abscess)

This occurs when infection spreads through the tonsil capsule into the potential space between capsule and tonsil bed. The resulting accumulation of pus is usually antero-superior to the tonsil, just behind the anterior faucial pillar. The complication is rare before the age of 12 years.

Increasing unilateral throat pain develops a few days after the onset of tonsillitis. Pain becomes severe, radiating into the ear, with trismus and drooling. The patient is feverish and toxic, and tries to avoid swallowing. Gross unilateral swelling is obvious on examination of the pharynx.

Treatment. In the early stages, it may be possible to bring about resolution by means of penicillin injections (Benzylpenicillin 0.6 g 6-hourly intramuscularly for adults, half this dose in children aged 5–12 years).

For established quinsies, where appearances indicate presence of pus near the surface, incision gives immediate relief. General anaesthesia is not required and incision may be undertaken in the outpatient department, or occasionally in the surgery or patient's home, using a scapel blade (e.g. size 15 Bard-Parker) round which adhesive tape has been wrapped so that only 0.5 cm of the tip is uncovered. Incision is made into the most prominent part of the swelling after application of local anaesthetic (such as xylocaine spray). The patient is seated for the procedure and holds a basin into which the drained pus is spat. Sinus forceps should be thrust into the incision and opened to encourage drainage.

Since quinsy is such a painful condition, and has a strong tendency to recure, tonsillectomy 2 or 3 months later is often advised.

Consequences of adenotonsillar hyperplasia

Lymphoid hyperplasia, largely in response to infection, leads to enlargement of the tonsils and adenoids normally maximal around the age of 5 years. This enlargement, usually symptomless, is sometimes sufficient to cause inconvenience, and occasionally gross enough to be life-threatening. Whether energetic treatment of acute tonsillitis lessens the incidence of gross hypertrophy is uncertain.

Adenoidal hypertrophy and Eustachian ventilation

Adenoidal enlargement was formerly held to be an important cause of Eustachian obstruction. Disappointing results following adenoidectomy have thrown considerable doubt on this.

Cor pulmonale due to gross adenotonsillar hypertrophy

The potential threat to life posed by grossly enlarged tonsils and adenoids has only become widely appreciated during the last 20 years. In the USA in 1966, Luke et al reported cases of four children with severe respiratory difficulty resulting from enlarged tonsils and adenoids. All had cardiac enlargement and were cured by adenotonsillectomy. ECG changes before and after operation are shown in Fig. 13.2. By 1974 during one 12-month period, Jaffee was able to collect five cases of cor pulmonale, pulmonary hypertension, and congestive cardiac failure all corrected by removal of tonsils and adenoids. He suggested that less severe but damaging degrees of obstruction must be common. In the UK Freeland (1981) examined the ECGs of 95 unselected children awaiting tonsillectomy. Three showed right atrial hypertrophy with tall T waves, corrected by operation. Elevated arterial CO_2 concentration has been demonstrated in a group of 14 children with sleep apnoea (lasting longer than 20 seconds in five) using the non-invasive technique of capnography where a thin catheter is placed in the nose or mouth and end-expiratory CO_2 pressure in equilibrium with arterial pCO_2, is continuously monitored (Lind & Lundell, 1982). All showed elevated CO_2 pressure when awake and this increased greatly during sleep. All had normal ECGs, chest X-rays, and haematocrit values. (Nine children had already undergone adenoidectomy.) In all, tonsillectomy was followed by normalisation of arterial CO_2 pressure, and attacks of sleep apnoea ceased. All showed a subsequent significant increase in growth rate.

Clinical picture

Children with severely enlarged tonsils and adenoids breathe noisily during sleep, with periods of apnoea. They are often irritable and drowsy and perform poorly at school. Additional features reported in affected children included enuresis, facial oedema, obesity or underweight (major releases of growth hormone occur during REM sleep) hepatomegaly and polycythemia.

Recognition

With the declining popularity of adenotonsillectomy, serious upper airway obstruction due to enlarged tonsil and airways can be expected to become more common, and recognition falls to the gen-

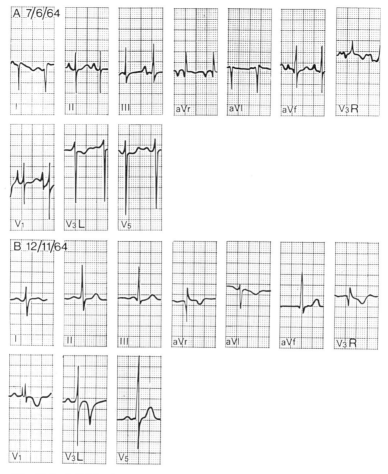

Fig. 13.2. A ECG of FF on 6 July 1964 one day after emergency admission. Note peaked P waves of right atrial hypertrophy in leads II and VI, right axis deviation and right ventricular hypertrophy. B ECG on 11 December 1964, four months after tonsillectomy and adenoidectomy, shows resolution of the hypertrophy pattern.

eral practitioner. It is important to identify not only the extreme cases with ECG abnormalities in whom continuing obstruction may be fatal, but also the less severely obstructed children in whom permanent damage to mental and physical development may result. Serious obstruction is indicated by noisy breathing at night, with episodes of sleep apnoea. The parents should always be questioned regarding the occurrence of sleep apnoea, and where doubt exists a home visit in the evening may be called for: sometimes a tape recording of breathing during sleep is helpful. (Snoring without apnoea attacks appears to be harmless.)

Inspection of the throat will reveal gross tonsillar hypertrophy, the medial surfaces being flattened by contact in the midline.

Treatment

Tonsillectomy is imperative, as a matter of urgency, once severe obstruction has been recognised. Inclusion of the child's name on a waiting list is inappropriate and potentially lethal.

TONSILLECTOMY

Few subjects in medical care have caused so much controversy as tonsillectomy. The operation has a long history: Cornelius Celsus described a technique in the first century. During the first half of the present century tonsillectomy (often with adenoidectomy) was extensively undertaken for a wide range of indications. Some children died as the result of unnecessary tonsillectomy (the operation still carries a mortality of about 1 in 25 000) but a great number of children benefited from the operation. During the 1960s, thanks largely to the observations of Fry (1966) from his general practice, the natural history of tonsillitis became better understood. Fry highlighted the peak incidence of tonsillitis in children aged 5–6 years, with a rapid reduction in attack rate thereafter. Wider appreciation of the self limiting tendency of recurrent tonsillitis, and increasing awareness of the immunological role of the tonsils and adenoids resulted in a declining demand for adenotonsillectomy. Between 1967 and 1973 the number of adenotonsillectomy operations in Scotland dropped by 40% (from 28 225 to 17 049) and in England and Wales, by 1977 the operation rate had fallen by over 50% (to 100 460). The most recent DHSS figures (1981) indicated just over 71 000 operations annually.

Indications for tonsillectomy

Wood's (1973) criteria for advising tonsillectomy are widely accepted.

1. *Repeated attacks of tonsillitis* after scrutiny of school record, attack rate, throat swab and serum IgA determination. 25 per cent

of children suffering from recurrent sore throats have a deficiency of IgA and can be expected to continue to have sore throats whether or not their tonsils are removed (Donovan & Soothill, 1973).

2. Quinsy (p. 191).

3. Recurrent tonsillitis with otitis media as in 1.

4. Evidence of chronic streptococcal infection (especially where acute rheumatism has occurred).

5. Gross obstruction of the air passages.

Repeated attacks of tonsillitis as an indication for tonsillectomy

Attempts to specify a frequency of attacks of tonsillitis to be judged as indicating the need for tonsillectomy are not helpful. Paradise (1978) followed up for 1 year 65 children with at least seven episodes of throat infection in 1 year, five in each of 2 consecutive years, or three in each of 3 years. He found that 43 experienced either no further infections or at the most only one or two infections, mostly mild. Only 11 conformed to the previously reported pattern.

The limited value of throat swabs in view of wide discrepancies between surface and core tonsil bacteriology, has already been noted (p. 190).

Economic considerations

These may influence the decision to advise tonsillectomy for a child with recurrent tonsillitis. His mother may be the bread winner, and her job may be jeopardised by frequent absences from work when he is ill with tonsillitis. Unfortunately such children are liable to be taken late for treatment, and are therefore prone to chronic tonsil infection.

The greater severity of tonsillitis in adults, and tendency to recur indefinitely, increases the place for tonsillectomy in this age group.

The importance of indication 5. (gross obstruction of the air passages) is increasingly recognised (p. 193).

Indications for adenoidectomy

Enlarged adenoids referred for surgery are usually curetted along with dissection of the tonsils at one operation.

Owing to the strong tendency for remaining elements of Waldeyer's ring to hypertrophy if a portion is removed, removal of adenoids alone is all too often followed by considerable enlargement of the tonsils, calling for a second operation. Banham (1968) surveyed 1000 school leavers who had undergone tonsillectomy, and advised 'If the adenoids warrant removal the tonsils are similarly infected and should be removed at the same time'.

Adenoidectomy has traditionally been advocated to benefit middle ear problems by relieving Eustachian obstruction. It seems unlikely however that enlarged adenoids are an important cause of Eustachian obstruction. In one investigation (Hibbert & Stell, 1982) the size of adenoids in a series of children with middle ear fluid was compared radiologically with a series of age and sex matched children with no fluid. There was no significant difference. As Sadé (1979) comments 'Only a large scale, preferably prospective study, could demonstrate conclusively whether adenoidectomy has any minor therapeutic effect or none at all'.

The general practitioner's role in the management of tonsil and of adenoid problems

Summary

1. Prompt treatment of acute tonsillitis with antibiotics offers the best hope of preventing chronic infection and severe hypertrophy. General practices should be organised so that treatment is readily available.

2. Parents often benefit from an explanation of the natural history of tonsil and adenoid problems, and the principles of modern management. They are then better able to co-operate in the plan of tiding the child over the difficult 4–6-year age period, after which spontaneous improvement can be expected. They are also more likely to rely on their doctor, aware of the extent of morbidity, to judge in consultation if and when tonsillectomy is called for, rather than to feel they must demand surgery.

3. The general practitioner must be constantly alert for symptoms and signs of serious adenotonsillar obstruction, including sleep apnoea (p. 193).

4. As is so often true, the best patient care results when general practitioner and specialist know each other well enough to co-operate closely.

REFERENCES

Banham T M 1968 A survey of 1000 school leavers who have had their tonsils removed. Journal of Laryngology and Otology 82:203

Brook I, Yocum P, Shah K 1980 Surface v core tonsillar aerobic and anaerobic flora in recurrent tonsillitis. Journal of the American Medical Association (15): 1696–1698

Donovan R, Soothill J F 1973 Immunological studies in children undergoing tonsillectomy.

Editorial 1983 Penicillin for sore throats. The Practitioner. 227 (1386):891

Freeland A 1981 Airway obstruction from adenotonsillar hypertrophy. British Medical Journal 282: 1579–1581

Fry J 1966 Profiles of disease. Churchill Livingstone; London

Hibbert J, Stell P M 1982 The role of enlarged adenoids in the aetiology of serous otitis media. Clinical Otolaryngology 7: 253–256

Jaffee I S 1974 Adenotonsillectomy as the treatment of serious medical conditions: five case reports. The Laryngoscope 84:1135

Kyeton J F, Pillsbury H C, Saskic T 1982 Nasal obstruction. Adenoiditis v adenoid hypertrophy. Archives of Otolaryngology 108: 315–318

Lind M G, Lundell B P W 1982 Tonsillar hyperplasia in children. Archives of Otolaryngology 108: 650–654

Luke M J, Mehrizi A, Folger G M, Rowe R D 1966 Chronic nasopharygeal obstruction as a cause of cardiomegaly, cor pulmonale and pulmonary oedema. Pediatrics 37:762

Paradise J L 1978 History of recurrent sore throat as an indication for tonsillectomy. Preditive limitations of histories that are undocumented. New England Journal of Medicine 298 (8): 405–412

Sadé J 1979 In: Secretory otitis media and its sequelae. Churchill Livingstone London p 269

Saski C T, Koss N 1978 Chronic baterial tonsillitis. Fact or fiction? Oto laryngologic Clinics of North America 86: 854–864

Wood C B S 1973 Tonsillectomy. The Practitioner 211:713

14

Croup and hoarseness

CROUP

The susceptibility of infants to noisy breathing and a barking cough, 'croup', in the presence of upper respiratory infection results from the following.

1. The small size of the infant larynx.
2. Poor immunity to many viruses and bacteria.
3. The presence of plentiful loose submucous areolar tissue in the infant larynx, especially at the laryngeal inlet and in the subglottic region. Considerable oedema and inflammatory infiltration readily occur.
4. The especially brisk nature of reflex responses in infancy, with a consequent enhanced tendency to laryngeal spasm.

Minor degrees of laryngeal obstruction, from simple viral laryngitis, commonly accompany upper respiratory tract infections in babies and young children. There is often merely a gruffness of the voice, and a hoarse barking cough, with little fever or malaise. Most cases clear up in 1 or 2 days and no special treatment is needed. If constitutional upset is marked, or the symptoms prolonged, secondary bacterial infection may be suspected and an antibiotic (such as penicillin V) prescribed. 'Soothing' linctuses, such as paediatric simple linctus BP, are popular.

More severe episodes of croup typically occur at night. Loud stridorous breathing usually alerts the parents to the infant's distress. The instinct is to lift him, sit him on a knee, console him, and send for the doctor. By the time the doctor arrives the breathing difficulty has often lessened although the stridor continues. This improvement may be attributed to the following:

1. Being brought down from a cold bedroom to the comforting warmth of the living room.
2. Parental consolation reducing the infant's disposal to cry.
3. The upright position encouraging laryngeal oedema to subside.

Every effort should be made to prevent crying, since this will increase laryngeal oedema. Examination should be as unobtrusive as possible: the clinical picture seldom leaves the diagnosis much in doubt. Steam is usually very effective in relieving croup, and can be obtained in the bathroom by turning on a hot shower, or in the kitchen by boiling water in saucepans. Laryngitis may be a painful condition and a small dose of aspirin may be helpful. Antibiotic treatment (penicillin V or amoxycillin) should be started if pyrexia is present. Before leaving the house, once breathing is easy, it is important to explain the need to report any subsequent deterioration in breathing: hospital admission may then be needed.

The presence of indrawing of the soft tissues of the root of the neck and thorax is a most significant warning sign that a potentially dangerous degree of respiratory obstruction exists, calling for hospital facilities.

Severe croup may complicate measles, particularly in developing countries where mortality is high. Laryngeal obstruction with respiratory and cardiac arrest contributes to this mortality.

Croup in diphtheria is almost invariably accompanied by faucial involvement.

Acute epiglottis

This condition occurs most often in boys aged 2–4 years, but may occur in either sex in children and adults. Mortality rates of up to 50 % have been reported. Onset is rapid: a fit child may be in dire distress within 6 hours. Initially there is usually a sore throat, then difficulty in swallowing, drooling, retching, and difficulty in breathing. There is usually high fever. Stridor, hoarseness and croupy cough are often absent, as the inflammatory changes are above the glottis.

Acute epiglottitis is usually a local manifestation of a capsulated *Haemophilus influenzae* type B bacteraemia, and blood culture is more likely to reveal the organism than a throat swab.

The epiglottis is bright red, swollen and boggy, but the main airway obstruction usually results from swelling of the false cords (many consider 'supraglottitis' would be a better term).

Children with acute epiglottitis often adopt a characteristic position, sitting up in a tripod fashion with arms and head back, mouth opened, and the jaw protroding.

Treatment of acute epiglottis

Establishment of an airway is urgently required. The general practitioner confronted by a child with suspected epiglottitis in extreme respiratory distress and far from a hospital should never attempt to visualise the epiglottis: introduction of a tongue depressor may well trigger cardiac arrest. Probably the best emergency treatment is to introduce one or more intravenous needles of the widest available bore direct into the trachea.

In adults in great emergency, laryngotomy (p. 206) is probably the best course.

Once in hospital, children are managed with positive pressure ventilation whilst an expert intubationist is summoned. At intubation the diagnosis is confirmed by direct laryngoscopy, and a swab of the epiglottis taken. Antibiotic treatment with intravenous ampicillin and chloromycetin (the latter since some strains of *H. influenzae* are resistant to ampicillin) is begun. Intubation is usually necessary for 3 days. Intravenous dexamethasone 1–1.5 mg/kg body weight is also given in many centres.

Adults reaching hospital are usually managed by tracheostomy.

Acute laryngo-tracheo-bronchitis

This condition occurs chiefly between the ages of 6 months and 3 years, again primarily affecting boys. Most cases occur in winter or spring.

Many viruses have been implicated. Parainfluenzae type 1 is the commonest cause, and para-influenzae type 2 the second most common. Respiratory syncitial virus is a less common cause.

Typically, during an upper respiratory tract infection a gradual inspiratory stridor develops, with hoarseness, a barking cough, and fever. Severe respiratory distress may develop after 3–7 days. There will then be a gross indrawing of soft tissues on inspiration, yet, in distinction from the picture in acute epiglottitis, the child is not disturbed by lying down.

Management

Urgent hospital admission is called for. If diagnosis in in any doubt, direct laryngosopy under general anaesthesia should be performed. In acute laryngo-tracheo-bronchitis there is severe destruction of ciliated epithelium, inflammatory exudate and oedema. Other possibly unsuspected causes for respiratory distress, such as a foreign body, can be excluded. A bronchoscope may be introduced and debris aspirated from the lower respiratory tract.

The patient is ideally nursed in a 'croupette' providing cool moist air with an ultrasonic atomiser. Oxygen and intravenous fluids may be needed. Racemic adrenaline aerosols administered by intermittent positive pressure breathing are sometimes used. Antibiotics and steroids are of doubtful value.

In cases deteriorating despite treatment, intubation and regular suction will be required. Intubation carries a serious risk of subsequent subglottic stenosis, and if it appears likely to be needed for 1 week or more, tracheostomy is necessary to avoid this complication.

Stridor in infants

Other causes of stridor include the following:
Allergic oedema of the vocal cords.
Inhaled foreign bodies.
Laryngeal trauma, from birth injury or intubation injury.
Congential abnormalities of the larynx, including laryngeal stenosis.
Laryngomalacia (congenital laryngeal stridor): noisy breathing continues, especially during sleep, until the age of 4–5 years. Weight gain may be retarded. There is no specific treatment.
Vagal and recurrent laryngeal nerve paralysis, sometimes the result of vagus nerve stretching during difficult delivery.

Site of obstruction

Some guide as to the site of obstruction in stridor is provided by the timing.

a. Inspiratory stridor generally indicates obstruction at or above the vocal cords.
b. Expiratory stridor alone suggests a constriction below the cricoid.

c. Combined inspiratory and expiratory stridor is typical of constriction at the cricoid level.

HOARSENESS

In the adult larynx, voice changes are much more common than respiratory obstruction. Hoarseness results wherever a normal smooth vocal cord is not brought evenly and firmly into apposition with its fellow on phonation. This may result either from structural abnormalities of the cord or from disturbances of neuromuscular control.

Malignancy should always be thought of whenever hoarseness persists for more than 1 or 2 weeks. Intrinsic carcinoma of the vocal cords is eminently curable it detected early. Once spread has occurred, the prognosis is much less favourable.

Acute hoarseness

Short-lived hoarseness most commonly results from acute laryngitis, occuring during the course of an upper respiratory tract infection. Attempts to speak may be painful and for a time the voice may be completely lost. Treatment consists of voice rest, steam inhalations, and antibiotics where secondary infection is suspected.

Acute hoarseness may be caused by minor cord trauma from shouting, coughing, vomiting, inhaling irritant fumes, from a blow to the larynx, or by allergic swelling of the cords.

Chronic hoarseness

This is arbitrarily defined as a voice change lasting more than 3 weeks.
Causes include:
a. unresolved acute hoarseness and
b. Chronic laryngitis.

Persisting hyperaemia, hypertrophy, or oedema of the cords may result from voice abuse, smoking, prolonged inhalation of irritant fumes, dust, spirit consumption, or frequent coughing or vomiting.

Singers' nodes

These are a localised form of chronic laryngitis: hyperkeratosis develops at the junction of the anterior and middle thirds of the cord on each side. They develop in some people who use 'forced' voices or sing above the normal range.

Contact ulcers

These may develop as a result of vocal abuse, posteriorly at the point overlying the vocal process of the arytenoid.

Vocal cord polyps

These are the commonest cause of chronic hoarseness. They affect particularly men in their 40s who speak in a strident way with unnecessary tension.

Treatment of chronic laryngitis in general involves voice rest and elimination of irritating factors. Air humidfication and steam inhalations may be helpful. Voice abuse calls for the attentions of a speech therapist, who is often able to help not only by retraining voice production but by general counselling of the patient in a bid to help him relax. Innocent swellings of the cords may need removal under the operating microscope.

In children, multiple viral *laryngeal papillomata* are the commonest cause of chronic hoarseness. Repeated removal under the operating microscope may be needed. Sometimes the papillomata are extensive throughout the respiratory tract and life threatening. Laser surgery and interferon have also been used in treatment.

Myxoedema

This may present with hoarseness. The vocal cords have a characteristic 'boggy' appearance.

Tubercular laryngitis and acquired syphilis

These are nowadays rare causes of chronic hoarseness.

Vocal cord palsy

This may be due to a lesion anywhere along the pathway from the cerebral cortex to the terminal branches of the superior and recurrent laryngeal nerves. Because of its longer course the left recurrent laryngeal is the more frequently involved. Nerve conduction may be interfered with as a result of spread of local disease (such as a bronchial carcinoma), trauma (particularly during thyroid and carotid endarterectomy surgery), peripheral neuritis due to viral disease, or to radiotherapy. Often no cause for a cord palsy can be found.

The condition of a cord may be found to be one of the following.

1. Flabby due to paralysis of the cricothyroid muscle the 'tensor' of the cord) supplied by the external branch of the superior laryngeal nerve.
2. Fixed in the midline and failing to abduct on inspiration.
3. Lying in the 'cadaveric' or paramedian position, neither abducting on deep inspiration nor adducting on phonation. In the case of a unilateral lesion, the normal cord will cross the midline to meet its fellow on phonation.

Semon's law states that in a progressive recurrent laryngeal nerve lesion the abductors are paralysed before the adductors. Thus 2. above, may be a stage in progression toward 3. Some have reservations about Semon's law, considering the position adopted by the paralysed cord to be fortuitous.

Hoarseness as a result of unilateral cord palsy tends to improve spontaneously. Speech therapy may speed recovery. Voice production where the affected cord is flaccid in the cadaveric position is sometimes successfully treated by injection of teflon paste. Where both cords are paralysed in adduction, respiratory difficulty usually necessitates tracheostomy. Some cases regain partial cord movement after up to 2 years and it may then be possible to discard the tracheostomy. Otherwise a satisfactory airway may be restored by Woodman's cordopexy: the arytenoid is partially removed on one side and the cord hitched laterally to the thyroid cartilage.

Malignant disease of the larynx

Hoarseness is the commonest presenting symptom of laryngeal cancer, which accounts for about 2 % of all cancers and affects men roughly eight times more frequently than women. Squamous cell carcinoma is the commonest form. Tobacco, spirits, and prolonged vocal strain appear to the aetiological factors. Anatomically, laryngeal cancers can be glottic (arising on the vocal cord itself, usually the middle or anterior third) or supraglottic or subglottic (arising above or below the cord).

Glottic carcinoma. This is much the commonest, and is usually well differentiated. It produces hoarseness at an early age, resulting in the opportunity for early diagnosis whilst still confined to one cord. Here the prognosis is exceptionally good, with a 5-year survival rate of about 95 % after radiotherapy.

Supra-glottic and subglottic carcinomas. These carry a much worse prognosis. They tend not to produce symptoms untill well advanced, and spread early to lymph nodes in the neck.

ACUTE LARYNGEAL OBSTRUCTION

Causes of acute laryngeal obstruction include acute laryngotracheobronchitis (the commonest), acute epiglottitis, inflammatory oedema complicating quinsy, Ludwig's angina or retropharangeal abscess, laryngeal diphtheria, angioneurotic oedema, external trauma to the larynx with submucosal haemorrhge, and internal trauma from inhaled steam, fumes, or swallowed corrosives.

Most inhaled foreign bodies do not stick in the larynx, but pass down to the tracheal bifurcation or into the right main bronchus. However in children inhaled foreign bodies such as coins can lodge in the larynx: choking is the leading cause of accidental death in the home for infants under 1 year of age.

Choking leading to sudden death may occur during a meal, a large piece of steak partially entering the larynx where it is held by reflex spasm. Such incidents ('Cafe coronaries') have been mistakenly diagnosed as myocardial infarctions.

Treatment of acute laryngeal obstruction

Where obstruction from a foreign body is strongly suspected, the 'Heimlich manoeuvre' should be performed: positioned behind the victim the rescuer clasps his hands in the epigastrium and delivers repeated upwards thrusts to expel the impacted object.

For other cases *laryngotomy* is usually the best course. With the patient's head extended, the laryngeal cartilages are palpated and the gap between the thyroid and cricoid cartilage identified. A transverse incision (Fig. 14.1) is made over this gap using any knife or pair of scissors available, passing first through skin and next through the cricothyroid membrane. The cartilages are prised apart (possibly by rotating the knife blade) allowing the passage of air.

CROUP AND HOARSENESS 207

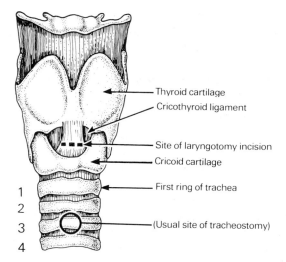

Fig. 14.1 Laryngotomy incision.

If any suitable tube, such as the barrel of a ball-point pen, is available it can be inserted to maintain the opening, otherwise the cartilages can be kept separated by the rotated knife blade. A council of perfection would be for every doctor to have in his bag a combined knife and laryngostomy tube (Cawthorne, 1964).

In infants, acute laryngeal obstruction may be relieved by insertion of a few needles of the widest available bore into the trachea.

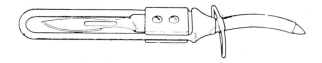

Fig. 14.2 Cawthorne emergency laryngostomy tube (scale 3/4)

REFERENCES

Cawthorne T 1964. Lancet 1081

15
Dysphagia

Introduction

Difficulty in swallowing is quite a common complaint in general practice. The symptom tends to be disquieting, for the possibility of an underlying malignant cause is often at the back of the mind of the patient, or doctor, or both.

Difficulty affecting the early stages of swallowing, passing the food bolus back to the throat and initiating the swallowing reflex, indicates a neuromuscular cause such as multiple sclerosis, motor neurone disease, bulbar palsy, or posterior cerebellar artery thrombosis. It is always worth seeking an ENT opinion in such cases for, providing that closure of the larynx is still possible, the operation of cricopharyngeal myotomy (in which the fibres of the cricopharyngeus are divided from an external approach) may greatly assist swallowing.

Acute dysphagia

This may result from swallowing of caustics, infections such as candidiasis, or following the swallowing of foreign bodies.

Emergency treatment of swallowed caustics consists of shock and pain relief, and neutralisation of the corrosive with appropriate oral weak acids or alkalis. Hospital admission is usually needed for intravenous fluids and antibiotics, and for tracheostomy if laryngeal oedema supervenes. The risk of subsequent stricture formation is lessened if a nasogastric tube is kept in place for 2 to 3 weeks. Careful follow-up, with repeated barium meal X-rays, is needed for 6 months once normal swallowing is resumed, so that incipient strictures can be recognised and dilated in good time.

Candidiasis of the pharynx and oesophagus, chiefly affecting debilitated patients, those on steroids, and following broad spectrum antibiotics, can cause very painful dysphagia. Treatment consists of Nystatin suspension given orally every 2–3 hours, and parenteral vitamins and fluid replacement where necessary. In severe cases a nasogastric feeding tube may be needed for a few days.

Foreign bodies

Coins, bones, open safety pins and lumps of meat are among the commoner objects to lodge in the throat.

Fish bones are particularly liable to stick in tonsillar crypts or at the base of the tongue. In the former position they may be more easy to feel with the finger than to see, and may be simply removed with angled forceps, pushed sideways during closure so that the fishbone protrudes from the crypt and can be grasped.

The oropharynx should be examined with a head mirror and spatula. A laryngeal mirror is required to examine the laryngopharynx. If the patient can lateralise the foreign body this indicates that it is above the level of the cricoid and should therefore be visible in a mirror. Most visible foreign bodies can be removed without recourse to a general anaesthetic. The patient's co-operation is essential: he must understand what is being done and helps by grasping his tongue in a gauze swab and pulling it forwards to improve the view. Holding a mirror in his left hand, the doctor guides a suitable pair of angled forceps down with his right hand until the foreign body can be grasped. Some foreign bodies are readily removed in the surgery by practitioners familiar with the use of a head mirror, but many will necessitate the services of a skilled laryngologist.

Referral to an ENT department will also be necessary for all patients in whom the presence of an unseen foreign body is suspected. Plain films of the neck and chest, followed where necessary by barium studies, may reveal the swallowed object, which can then be removed at oesophagoscopy. Some foreign bodies cannot be located until oesophagoscopy is performed.

Hiatus hernia

'Sliding' hiatus herniae often cause discomfort in the throat in addition to symptoms located in the lower retrosternal region. Throat symptoms may vary from vague discomfort to redness and soreness of the pharynx, with cricopharyngeal spasm and dysphagia. Discomfort in the throat, with difficulty in swallowing referred to the cricoid level, may be the presenting symptom of hiatus hernia: the diagnosis may be missed unless barium swallow X-ray or endoscopy is performed. Treatment with Gaviscon Gel and ranitidine usually relieves symptoms promptly. Stricture formation at the lower oesophagus, the end result of recurring reflux oesophagitis, is a difficult condition to treat. Thoracic surgeons are keen that patients with reflux oesophagitis not responding to medical management should be referred to them early, so that surgical repair can be undertaken before the development of fibrosis and constriction.

Achalasia cardia

This condition, most common in men between 30 and 60 years of age, appears to result primarily from degeneration of ganglion cells in Auerbach's plexus at the lower end of the oesophagus; although changes higher in the oesophagus, and in the vagi, have been described. The cause is unknown.

Initially there is merely epigastric discomfort, followed by the onset of dysphagia, the severity of which tends to wax and wane for many months. Eventually regurgitation develops.

Barium swallow X-ray demonstrates dilatation of the oesophagus above the obstruction, and, in later cases, lack of peristalsis associated with atrophy of the oesophageal musculature.

Oesophagoscopy is necessary to establish the diagnosis and exclude an underlying neoplasm. Many cases are managed by repeated dilatation with bougies, or other instruments. Alternatively Heller's operation of cardiomyotomy gives good results.

Pharyngeal pouch

This is a posterior herniation of the wall of the laryngopharynx through Killian's dehiscence, a weakened area in the inferior constrictor between the cricopharyngeus below and the thyropharyngeus above. Although the neck of the pouch is near the midline posteriorly, the fundus usually presents as a swelling on the left side of the neck. There is long-standing and increasing dysphagia, with regurgitation of undigested food. Pressure over the pouch may result in gurgling and emptying.

Barium swallow X-ray outlines the contours of the pouch. Small pouches may need no treatment, or the symptoms may be relieved by cricopharyngeal myotomy. External excision of larger pouches is usually curative. For frail and debilitated patients Dohlman-type operations, in which the tissues separating the lumen of the pouch from the lumen of the oesophagus are destroyed by diathermy, are less traumatic.

Sideropenic dysphagia (Paterson Brown-Kelly or Plummer-Vinson syndrome)

In this condition iron deficiency leads to atrophic changes in the mucosa of the upper alimentary tract predisposing to mechanical, chemical, and heat trauma from food. Clinically this tends to be most obvious on the lips and tongue: angular stomatitis and glossitis are common. The mucosa of the upper oesophagus and post-cricoid area is particularly susceptible and the resulting inflammation causes dysphagia. Webs or strictures may develop.

The condition is much commoner in women and is particularly likely to complicate hiatus hernia with oesophagitis or to follow partial gastrectomy. It usually responds to administration of iron and prompt treatment is important, not only to control symptoms but because post-cricoid carcinoma may develop. In one series (Richards, 1970) of 266 patients with post-cricoid carcinoma, 35% had had dysphagia for more than 5 years at the time of diagnosis.

Globus hystericus

In this condition the patient, often a middle aged woman, complains of the sensation of a lump in the throat, usually in the region of the thyroid cartilage. Frequent attempts to swallow the lump may be made, aggravating the symptoms and leading to aerophagy and gastric discomfort. The symptoms improve or disappear whilst eating meals. A reason for anxiety, such as recent death of a friend from cancer of the throat is often present.

The general practitioner can hardly reassure the patient merely on negative clinical examination and without investigation. A negative barium swallow may suffice, but if symptoms continue referral for oesophagoscopy will be needed.

The symptoms in some cases will prove to be associated with cricopharyngeus spasm, secondary to an unsuspected hiatus hernia.

When barium studies and endoscopy are normal, a little time spent with the patient discussing the throat as a common target site for the emotions, and sympathetic consideration of some of her anxieties, is often more helpful than the prescription of tranquillisers.

Carcinoma of the laryngo-pharynx and oesophagus

1. Laryngo-pharynx

The pyriform fossa is the commonest site of carcinoma of the laryngo-pharynx. Men in their sixth and seventh decades are predominantly affected. Tobacco and alcohol appear to play an important part in aetiology and pipes and cigars may be more dangerous here than cigarettes. Owing to the relatively greater width of the food passage at this point, tumours may become large before dysphagia develops, and the disease may present with a palpable lymph node in the neck and pain referred to the ear. Hoarseness may develop as a result of local spread.

The post-cricoid region is the next commonest site of laryngo-pharyngeal carcinoma, and is seen almost exclusively in women, sometimes as young as 30 years, who have suffered from sideropenic dysphagia (p. 211). They may already have required dilatation of post-cricoid webs. Obstructive difficulties occur early, fluids being swallowed more easily than solids. Pain is not common in the early stages.

Pyriform fossa tumours should be visible with a laryngeal mirror. The post-cricoid region is beyond the field of view with a mirror, but frothy mucus collects in the pyriform fossa indicating obstruction beyond.

Management

Ideally, patients with suspected laryngo-pharyngeal carcinoma should be referred to an ENT department at a centre where radiotherapy is available, since this will usually be employed in treatment.

Most patients are treated initially with radiotherapy alone. Subsequent close follow-up is essential, and exacting, since recurrence of disease requiring further radiotherapy, or surgery, is difficult to detect at an early and still treatable stage.

The prognosis in laryngo-pharyngeal carcinoma is poor. In one series of patients (76 so far) who have come to laryngo-pharyngectomy the overall 5-year survival rate is only 22.2%. However in the 24 patients referred for surgery before lymph node involvement was detectable, this figure is improved to 55%. (Slaney & Dalton, 1983).

2. Oesophagus

Carcinoma of the oesophagus occurs most commonly in men over the age of 50 years. Tobacco, alcohol, reflux oesophagitis, and achalasia, are recognised predisposing factors. Symptoms are often delayed until the tumour is advanced and inoperable. Dysphagia, once established is rapidly progressive and obstruction may suddenly become complete as a result of impaction of a piece of food.

A high index of suspicion in general practice and early referral for barium swallow or oesophagoscopy offers the best hope of cure. For carcinomas of the middle and lower thirds of the oesophagus, oesophagectomy in the hands of a thoracic surgeon may be feasible. For most patients, especially where there is involvement of the bronchial tree, or recurrent laryngeal nerve, or distant metastases, palliative measures alone are available. Tumour regression may be achieved with radiotherapy. An indwelling tube (such as Owen's) may be inserted through the tumour region with an oesophagoscope to maintain a passage for feeding. A flange at the upper end of the tube prevents it from passing downwards. Patients eat a well liquidised diet washed down with copious fluids.

REFERENCES

Richards S H 1970 Post-cricord carcinoma in the Paterson Brown-Kelly syndrome. Journal of Laryngology 85: 141–152
Slaney G, Dalton G A 1983 Pharyngeal reconstruction by colonic transposition grafts. In: Bevan P G (ed) Reconstructive procedures in surgery. Blackwell Scientific Publications, London, p 67–86

Index

Abscess
  cerebellar, 52, 53
  extradural, 38, 39, 52, 53
  retropharyngeal, 206
  subdural, 52
  temporal lobe, 53
Achalasia cardia, 210, 213
ACTH, 155
Acoustic feedback ('whistling)', 116
Acoustic impedence, 43
Acoustic neuroma, 77, 96, 103, 123, 126
  brain-stem evoked responses in, 78, 79
Action potential
  in auditory pathway, 77
  from displaced basilar membrane, 78
  in vestibular nerve, 125
Acute labyrinthitis, see Failure, sudden vestibular
Adenoidectomy, 45, 178, 192, 193, 195
  indications for, 196–197
Adenotonsillar enlargement, see Hyperplasia, adenotonsillar
Adenotonsillar hypertrophy, see Hyperplasia, adenotonsillar
Adenotonsillectomy, 178, 179, 193, 195
Adenoids, 41, 137, 140, 175, 176, 177, 191
Adenoviruses, 139, 186
Adhesions (nasal), 162
Aditus, 26
Adrenergic blocking agents, 161
Adrenoceptor stimulants, 155
Adrenaline
  injection B D, 156–157
  racemic aerosols, 202
Advisory Committee on Services for Hearing Impaired People (ACSHIP), 108, 110

Aerophagy, 211
Age/sex register, 82
Air-bone gap, 88, 90
Air conduction, 72
Alcohol, 154, 205, 213
Alkali phosphatase, 41
Allergic perennial rhinitis, 157
Allergy (atopy), 40, 41, 45, 92, 152, 153
American Tinnitus Association, 124
Amikacin, 34
Aminoglycosides, 33, 34, 86, 103
Aminophylline injection BP, 157
Amoxycillin, 34, 35, 142, 146, 191, 200
Ampicillin, 146, 191, 201
Anaerobic commensuals, 143, 144
Anaerobic organisms see Organisms, anaerobic
Angina
  Ludwig's, 206
  Vincent's 188
Angled forceps, 9, 167
Anosmia, 141, 143, 164
Anoxia, foetal, 81
Antarctic, 138
Anterior nares, 133
Antibiotics, 49, 60, 142, 149, 203, 209
  in acute dysphagia, 208
  in acute laryngo-tracheo bronchitis, 202
  in croup, 199, 200
  prophylaxis, 37
  in tonsillitis, 189–191
Antibody, 31
  manufacture of, 178
Anticholinesterase drugs, 161
Anticoagulant therapy, 165
Antigen, 156, 178
Antihistamines, 45, 154, 155, 156, 162
  sedative side-effects, 154

INDEX

Antihypertensive drugs, 161
Antimicrobial agents
   mechanism of action, 34
   toxic reactions, 33
Antitoxin, diphtheria, 189
Antiviral agents, 142
Antral puncture, 148, 149
Antro-choanal polyp, 148, 163, 164
Antrum
   mastoid, 26, 28
   maxillary, *see* Sinuses, maxillary
Anxiety, 95
Aqueduct, cochlear, 66
Arctic, 138
Arteriosclerosis, 86
Arteriosclerotic patients, 165, 166
Arteries
   anterior ethmoid, 169
   anterior inferior cerebellar, 68
   basilar, 68
   external carotid, 169
   internal auditory, 103
   labyrinthine, 68, 127
   vertebral, 68, 103
Ashley, Mr Jack, 124
Aspirin, 35, 142, 147, 191
Astemizole (hismanal), 154
Asthma, 156
Atrophic sinusitis, 147
Attic, 27
Attico-antrostomy, 56
Atticotomy, 55
Audiogram
   normal, 76
   in Menière's disease, 94
   in noise induced hearing loss, 97, 98
   in otosclerosis, 88, 90
   in presbycusis, 106
   see also, 104, 122
Audiometer, 43, 50, 74, 100
   uses in general practice, 74
Audiometry, 36, 74
   method, 75
   Békésy, 77
   brain-stem electric response, 77
   electric (evoked) response, 77
   inpedence, 43
   in special centres, 77
Auditory pathway, 70, 77
Auditory response cradle, 83
Auroscope, *see* Otoscope
Automatic gain control, 115

Babbling, 80
Bacillus
   fragilis, 34
   Klebs-Loffler, 189
   melaninogenicus, 34
   Vincent's fusiform, 118
Bacteria
   anaerobic, 190
   commensual, 186
Batteries, 112, 115–116, 118
Bat ear, 18
Beales P.H., 90
Beclomethasone spray (Beconase), 155, 162, 164
Beconase, *see* Beclomethasone spray
Benign paroxysmal positional vertigo, 127, 128
Bernouilli phenomenon, 163
Betahistine (Serc), 95, 123
Beta-lactamase producers, 191
Betamethasone (Betnesol), 155
Birth injuries, 81
Bismuth iodoform paraffin paste (BIPP), 166
Blast injury, 97
Blindness, 108
Blocking antibody, 156
Blood culture, 200
Blood dyscrasias, 189
Blue steroid card, 155
Body worn aids, 109, 111
Bone conduction aids, 115
Bone conduction, 72
   measurement, 76
Brain-stem electric response
   audiometry, 77, 78, 79, 82, 94
   waves in, 78
Breast fed infants, 153
Brighton inflatable tampon, 166
Brill, G.C., 127
British Association of the Hard of Hearing, 120
British Association of Otolaryngologists, 101
British Deaf Association, 120
British Telecom, 119
British Tinnitus Association, 124
Bronchiolitis, 140
Bronchitis, 134
Bronchospasm, 153, 157
Budesonide (Rhinocort), 155
Bulb, inflation, 9, 10, 42, 54

Cacosmia, 143, 148
'Cafe coronaries', 206
Caldwell-Luc operation, 149
Caloric tests, 94, 123
Canal
   facial, 53

Canal (Cont'd)
  semicircular, 63, 64
  lateral, 27
Canaliculus, cochlear, 66
Candidiasis, 208, 209
Carbamazepine, 123
Carbenicillin, 33
Carbon dioxide (CO_2) concentration, 136
  arterial, 193
S-Carboxymethylcysteine (Mucodyne, Mucolex), 49
Carcinoma
  basal cell, 17
  bronchial, 205
  of laryngo-pharynx, 212
  of oesophagus, 213
  post-cricoid, 211, 212
  secondary, 103
  of vocal cords, 203, 205, 206
Carhart's notch, 88
Cartilages, laryngeal
  arytenoid, 179, 180, 204, 205
  corniculate, 179
  cricoid, 179, 180, 181, 202, 203, 206, 209
  cuneiform, 179
  epiglottis, 179, 180, 181
  thyroid, 179, 181, 205, 206, 211
Catarrh, nasal, 152
Catecholamine-depleting agents, 161
Caustics (for cauterisation), 169
Cauterisation (of the nose), 169
Ceefax, 119
Cells
  goblet, 31, 41, 134, 135
  fibroblasts, 178
  lymphocyte, 41, 175, 177, 178
  B & T lymphocytes, 153
  macrophage, 41, 178
  plasma, 178
  secretory, 41, 134
Cellulitis, 149
Celsus, Cornelius, 195
Central auditory pathway, 70, 104, 106, 107
Cephalosporins, 33
  cefaclor, 35, 146
  cephaloridine, 33
Chemotoxins, 153
Child development assessment clinics, 84
Childhood delinquency, 42
Chloramphenicol (chloromycetin), 33, 34, 86, 201

Chlorhexidine, 86
Chlorine, 144
Chlorpromazine (Largactil), 95, 127
Cholesteatoma, 36, 50, 51, 52, 53, 54, 56, 102
  congenital, 53
Chondrodermatitis nodularis chronicis helis, 17
Chromium trioxide, 169
Cilia, 134, 135, 136
  ciliary action, 31, 41, 135
  ciliated cells, 134
Cinnarizine (Stugeron), 95, 128
Clarinetists, 99
Clindamycin, 33, 34, 191
Cloxacillin, 191
Cochlea, 27, 63, 64, 66, 67, 93, 97, 101, 104, 105
  coils of, 81
Cochleostomy, 96
Code of practice, 110
Combined oral contraceptive, 91
Common cold, see Coryza
Complement fixation tests, 141
Complement, 41
Congestive cardiac failure, see Failure, congestive cardiac
Conjunctivae, 153
Conjunctivitis, 157
Cordopexy, woodman's, 205
Cords
  false, 180, 181, 184, 201
  vocal (true), 180, 181, 182, 185, 203
Contact ulcers, 204
Cor pulmonale, 193
Corti
  organ of, 66, 69, 106
  pillars of, 67
  tunnel of, 67
Corticosteroids (steroids), 36, 45, 103–104, 123, 155
Cortilymph, 67
Corynebacterium, diphtheriae, 189
Coryza (common cold), 29, 138–142, 143
Co-Trimoxazole, 34, 41, 146
Cough, and perilymph leak, 102
Crest, suprameatal, 28
Crista, 65
Cross infection, 138, 139
Croup, 199–200
Croupette, 202
Crypts, tonsil, 177, 209
Cupola, 65, 128
Cystic fibrosis, 163

Cytomegalovirus, 81
Cytotoxic drugs, 86

DDT, 136
Dead ear, 90
Deafness, 63–120
  in acute otitis media, 32
  in blast injury, 99
  incidence, 70
  investigation in consulting room, 72
  management, 110
  memory deficits in, 71
  in Menière's disease, 94
  from music, 99
  in noise induced hearing loss, 98
  in otitic barotrauma, 60
  problems within the family, 108
  problems at work, 109
  recognition, 71
  in traumatic tympanic membrane rupture, 59
  types, 71
    cochlear ('sensory'), 71, 77
    conductive, 71, 88, 112
    mixed, 71
    retrocochlear (neural), 71, 77
    sensorineural ('perceptive'), 71, 77, 85, 88, 90, 94
Deafness in childhood, 84–86
  causes, 85
  education, 85–86
Deafness in infancy
  causes, 80
  delay in provision of hearing aid, 80
  importance of early recognition, 80
  prevention, general practitioner's role, 81
  recognition, 82
  screening, 82–83
Decongestants, 35, 45, 49, 60, 61, 142, 146, 149, 154, 155, 164
Dehiscence, Killian's, 210
Dehydrogenases, 41
Dental infection, 143
Depression, 108
Dermatophagoides farinae, 157
Dermatophagoides pteronyssinus, 157
Desensitising injections, *see* Hyposensitising injections
Deviated nasal septum, 144, 148, 149
Devices in the home (deaf aids), 118
Dexamethasone, *see* Steroids
Dextrocardia, 134
Diabetic neuropathy, 127
Dietician, 160

Dihydrostreptomycin, 103
Dimotapp, 35, 60, 147, 162
Diphtheria, 189, 200, 206
Disablement benefit for occupational deafness, 100
Discotheques, 99
Distortion, 117, 118
District health budget, 112
Diving, 144
Dizziness, 124–129
Drooling, 192, 200
Duct
  cochlear (scala media), 63–66, 69
  endolymphatic, 63, 64
Ductus reuniens, 63, 64
Dynein, 134, 135
Dyslexia, 42
Dysphagia, 209–213
  sideropenic (syn. Paterson Brown-Kelly or Plummer-Vinson syndrome), 221, 212

ENT teaching, 3
Ear, congenital malformation of, 18, 82
Ear drops, sodium bicarbonate, 21, 85
Ear level aids, 109, 113
Ear moulds, 113, 116
Earphones (hearing aid), 115
Ear plugs, 99
Ear protectors, 98, 99, 100, 110
Electric (evoked) response audiometry, 77, 94
Electrocardiograms (ECGs), 194
  in children awaiting tonsillectomy, 193
  in sleep apnoea, 193
Electrocautery, 168, 169
Electrocochleography, 77, 78, 94
Education of deaf children, 85–86
Embolism, of cochlear vessels, 86
Emergency tray, 156
Encephalitis, brain stem, 127
Endolymph, 63, 66, 68, 92, 96
  pressure, 95
Endolymphatic hydrops, 92
Enuresis, 193
Eosinophils, 163
Ephedrine, 155, 158
  nose drops, 136
Epidemic kerato-conjunctivitis, 139
Epiglottis, 138
  infantile, 185
Epiglottitis, acute, 200, 201, 206
Epilepsy, 126
Epistaxis, 148, 165–169

218 INDEX

Epithelial migration, 16, 22, 23, 25
Epithelium
  ciliated columnar, 26, 134
  cuboidal, 26
  squamous, 134
Erectile tissue, 160
Ergot preparations, 161
Erythromycin, 34, 86, 191
Esherichia coli, 34
Ethacrynic acid, 86, 103
Eustachian orifice (opening), 133, 137
Eustachian tube, 26, 28, 31, 50, 121, 123, 134, 175, 176
  eustachian obstruction, 41, 192, 197
  inadequate function, 58
Examination instruments
  ear, 8, 9, 10
  nose, 10, 11
  throat, 11
Exclusion diets, 159
Exostoses, cold water swimmers', 24

Failure
  congestive cardiac, 193
  sudden vestibular, 95, 127, 141
False negative Rinne test, 72, 88
Fenestration cavities, 88, 91
Fenestration operation, 69, 88, 89, 91
Fever, rheumatic, 190
  see also Rheumatism, acute
Fibroptic endoscopy, 137
Fistula
  labyrinthine, 50
  perilymph, 71, 90, 91
Fistula sign, 54
Fluctuating deafness (in Menières disease), 91
Fluid level (in sinus), 145
Flunisolide (Syntaris), 155
Fluorescent treponemal antibody test, 102
Fluoride, 90
Fold
  ary-epiglottic, 180, 181
  palatoglossal, 175
  palatopharyngeal, 175
Follicles, hair, 15
Food allergy, 157, 159–160
Forceps
  angled, 8, 9, 209
  crocodile, 8, 9, 24
  Quire's, 8, 9, 24
Foreign bodies
  in bronchus, 206
  in ear, 24
  in larynx, 182, 202, 206
  in pharynx and oesophagus, 208, 209
Fossa
  pyriform, 184, 212
  tonsillar, 188
Foxen, Miles, 52
Fracture, skull, 59
Frusemide, 86, 103
Fry, J., 29, 195
Fuller, A.P., 85
Furunculosis, 23, 38
Fusobacteria, 34

Ganglion
  spiral, 67
  submandibular, 27
  vestibular, 68
Gastro-intestinal (alimentary) tract, 140, 141
Gaviscon, 210
Gentamycin, 34, 103
Giddiness, 91, 92, 94
Glands
  ceruminous, 15
  sebaceous, 15
  salivary
    parotid, 28
    sublingual, 27
    submandibular, 27
Globus hystericus, 211
Glomerulonephritis, acute, 190
Glucose intolerance, 92
Glue ear (syn. secretory, serous, or 'non-suppurative' otitis media) 39–50, 58, 136
  aetiology, 40–42
  consequences, 42
  incidence, 39
  management, 45, 48–50
  natural history, 39
  recognition, 42
  screening for, 45
Glycerol dehydration, 94
Golgi apparatus, 135
Gradenigo's syndrome, 39, 53
Grass pollen, 40, 153
Greater London Association for the Disabled, 120
Gristwood, R.E., 53
Grommets, 45, 48, 49, 50, 61
  in Menière's disease, 95
  and swimming, 49
Growth in adenotonsillar hypertrophy, 193
Guanethidine (Ismelin), 161

H_1 receptors, 154
Haematoma, subperichondrial, 17
Haemaglobinopathies, 103
Haemophilus influenzae, 31, 34, 35, 37, 186
  type B, 200
Haemorrhage, 165
Hair cells, 65, 66, 67, 68, 70, 124
Hallpike and Cairns, 92
Hard-of-Hearing Medical Society, 120
Hay, 153
Hay fever, 152, 156
Head injury (trauma), 86, 92, 102, 126, 127, 128
Health and Safety Executive, 110
Health visitor, 83
Hearing, mechanism of, 68, 69, 70
Hearing aid, 58, 80, 91, 107, 109, 111–116, 124
  CROS, 117
  types, 113
Hearing aid amplifiers, 113, 115
Hearing aid clinics (centres), 109, 116
Hearing Aid Council, 112
Hearing Aid Industry Association, 112, 120
Hearing aid microphones, 113, 114
Hearing dogs for the deaf, 119
Hearing protectors, 98, 99
Hearing screening tests
  infants, 80, 82, 83, 84
  toddlers, 84
Hearing therapist, 110, 111
Helicotrema, 66, 67, 93
Helsinki declaration on medical ethics, 96
Heparin, 153
Hereditary deafness, 80, 86
Hereditary telangiectasia, 165, 169
Herpes zoster, 102
Hiatus hernia, 209–210, 211, 212
Hibitane, 86
High tone hearing loss, 104–107, 116
Higher education for deaf children, 86
Histamine, 153, 154, 156
Histamine drip, 103
Hoarseness, 201, 203–206, 212
Honeymoon rhinitis, 161
Housedust mite, 40, 157, 158
Hydrocortisone injection B P, 157
Hyperbilirubinaemia, 81
Hyperplasia (hypertrophy), adenotonsillar, 192
Hypertension, 123
  pulmonary, 193

Hypertrophy
  adenotonsillar, *see* Hyperplasia, adenotonsillar
  laryngeal, 203
  right antrial, 193
Hyposensitising ('desensitising') injections, 156–157
Hypotensive drugs, decongestants, 142, 155
Hypothalamus, 161
Hyposensitisation, 45
Hypotension, 167
Hypothyroidism, 92

Idiopathic sudden sensorineural deafness, 103
Imipramine, 162
Immune mechanisms, 133
Immunity, 138
Immunoglobulin
  lgA, 40, 41, 152, 153, 195, 196
  lgE, 40, 41, 152, 153, 156, 158–159
  lgG, 41, 156
  lgM, 41
Immunology
  immunological deficiency, 37
  type 3 immune complex, 40
Implant, cochlear, 71
Incus, 26, 27, 68
Induction coil, 113, 118
Induction loop, 109, 118, 119
Industrial compensation, 99
Industrial Injuries Advisory Council, 101
Inferior colliculus, 77
Infertility, 134
Ingested allergens, 159
Inhalations, 142, 147, 203, 204
Inner ear, 63–70
Insert (hearing aid), 113, 116
Institute of Hearing Research, 121
Interferon, 31, 142, 204
Internal auditory meatus, 68, 92
In-the-ear aids, 114
Intranasal antrostomy, 149
Intubation, 201, 202
  endotracheal tube, 182
Iron, 211
Islands of hearing, 80
Isoniazid, 33

Jordan, R., 39, 40
Jugular vein, 123
Juvenile angiofibroma, 165
Juvenile delinquency, 84

Kanamycin, 103
Kartagener's syndrome, 134
Karvol capsules, 147
Keratosis
  obturans, 25
  solar, 17
Kinocilium, 124
Klebsiella, 34

Labyrinth, 92, 124, 127
  bony, 63
  membranous, 63
Labyrinthine sedative, 128
Labyrinthectomy (destruction of labyrinth), 95
Labyrinthitis, 52, 102
Lamina, osseous spiral, 66
Lamp
  anglepoise, 7
  Chiron, 6, 7
  halogen, 6
  head worn, 6, 7, 183
  spirit, 12
Language aquisition, 80
Largactil (chlorpromazine), 95
Laryngitis, 141, 148
  chronic, 203–204
  syphilitic, 204
  tubercular, 204
Laryngomalacia (congenital laryngeal stridor), 202
Laryngopharynx, 175, 183
Laryngoscopy
  direct, 202
  indirect, 183–185
Laryngotomy, 201, 206
Laryngo-tracheo-bronchitis, acute, 140, 201, 202, 206
Larynx, 138, 179–185
Lateral lemniscus, 77
Leads, (hearing aid), 113, 118
Leukaemia, 86, 103, 165, 189
Life-threatening respiratory obstruction, 138
Ligament
  cricotracheal, 180
  spiral, 66
Ligation, arterial, 169
Linco-Bennett auditory response cradle, 83
Lincomycin, 33, 191
Link centre, 120
Lip reading, 71, 109, 111, 119, 120
Little's area, 165, 166
Local authority registers of deaf, 87
Lomusol (SCG), 156

Low frequency cut, 113, 115
Lower respiratory tract, 138, 141
Lozenge, benzocaine, 183
Lymphocytes, see Cells, lymphocyte
Lymphoid tissue, 134, 140, 175
  role of, 178–179
Lysozyme, 31, 41

Macewen's triangle, 28, 29, 38
Macroglobulinaemia, 103
Macrophages, 153
Macula
  of saccule, 66
  of utricle, 65
Malignant disease
  of larynx, 203, 205–206
  of oesophagus, 208
  of sinuses, 145
Malleus, 22, 27, 68
Malnutrition, 138
Manoevres
  Heimlich, 206
  Valsalva, 61
Masking, 72, 73, 75
Mast cells, 153, 155
Mastoidectomy, 45, 56, 58
  modified, 56, 57
  radical, 56, 57
  simple ('Schwartze'), 38, 57
Mastoidectomy cavities, 89
  aftercare, 56–58
Mastoiditis, 32, 52, 53
  acute, 38
  masked, 38
  zygomatic, 39
Maxillary ostium, 143
Maxillofacial anomalies, 81
Measles, 102, 200
Meatus, external auditory, 15, 16, 24, 25
  internal auditory, 68
Medical Board, 101
Medresco body worn aids, 112
Membrane
  basilar, 66, 69, 106
  cricothyroid, 206, 207
  Reissner's, 66, 67, 93
  Shrapnell's, 26
  tectorial, 66, 67
Menière, Prosper, 91
Menières disease, 91–96, 102, 123, 127
  clinical course, 94
  clinical picture, 94
  diagnosis, 94
  incidence, 92
  management, 95–96

Menières (Cont'd)
  transtympanic electrocochleogram in, 78
Menières syndrome, 92, 95
Meningitis, 39, 52, 53, 81, 86, 90, 103
Metaplasia
  (of middle ear mucosa in glue ear), 41
Methyldopa (Aldomet), 161
Methylprednisolone aqueous suspension (Depo-medrone), 155
Meati (of nose)
  inferior, 133, 134
  middle, 133, 163
  superior, 133, 134, 163
Microcomputers, 82
Microphone (hearing aid), 113, 117, 118
Microphonics, 69
Middle ear
  analyser, 43, 44, 45, 46–47
  anatomy, 26, 27, 28
  aspirates, 31, 40
  effusions, 31
Migen (Bencard), 160
Migraine, 92
Mirror
  head, 6, 7, 136, 183, 209
  laryngeal, 9, 12, 183, 209
Modiolus, 66
Monoamine oxidase inhibitor drugs, and decongestants, 142, 155
Mononucleosis, infectious, 188, 191
Motor neurone disease, 208
Mucociliary system, 134–136, 139, 143, 144, 146, 147, 164
Mucocoele of frontal sinus, 149, 150
Mycolytic agents, 45, 49
Mucus, 136
Mucus blanket, 134, 135
Mucus-secreting cells, 134
'Mulberry' turbinates, 160
Multiple sclerosis, 126, 127, 208
  brain-stem electric response audiometry in, 77
Mumps, 39, 85, 101
Muscles
  cricopharyngeus, 208, 210, 212
  cricothyroid, 180, 205
  intrinsic of larynx, 180
  levator palati, 41, 121
  stapedius, 26, 121
  superior constrictor, 177
  tensor tympani, 26, 121
  thyropharyngeus, 210
Myoclonic contractions, 121
Myotomy, cricopharyngeal, 208, 211
Myringitis, bullous (haemorrhagic), 25

Myringoplasty, 54, 55
Myringotomy, 35, 45, 50, 60
Myxoedema, hoarseness in, 204

Nasal airway cycle, 161
Nasal cavity, 133, 134, 138
Nasal deviation, 137
Nasal mucosa, 136, 153, 158, 166
Nasal obstruction, 148, 152, 154, 157, 161, 164
Nasal septum, 137
Nasal smears, 163
Nasal (silastic) splints, 162
Nasal vestibule, 134, 136
Nasopharynx, 133, 134, 138, 175
National Congenital Rubella Programme, 81
National Deaf Children's Society, 80, 120
Nausea and Vomiting, 91, 126, 127
Neisseria
  meningitidis, 34
  non-pathogenic, 191
Neomycin, 33, 103
Nephritis, 141
Nerve
  ampullary, 66, 68
  chorda tympani, 27
  cochlear, 68, 122
  eighth, 63, 96, 101, 122
  facial, 27
  glossopharyngeal, 28, 153
  lesser superficial petrosal, 28
  lingual, 27
  recurrent laryngeal, 180, 202, 204, 213
  saccular, 68
  superior laryngeal, 180, 204, 205
  tympanic, 28
  utricular, 68
  vagus, 180, 202, 210
    auricular branch, 19
  vestibular, 66, 68, 125
Nitrogen, absorption in middle ear, 41
Nitrogen mustard, 86
Nodes, lymph
  jugulo-digastric, 188
  posterior triangle, 188
Noise induced hearing loss, 97–101
Noisy occupations, 99
Non-allergic rhinitis, 152
Non-organic hearing loss, 77
Nose, 133–171
  anatomy, 133
  injuries, 170
Nucleus, cochlear, 77

Nystagmus, 94, 127, 128, 129
Nystatin, 209

Obstruction
  laryngeal, 206, 207
  Eustachian, see Eustachian obstruction
Oedema, angioneurotic, 206
Oesophagectomy, 213
Oesophagitis, 210, 213
Oesophagoscopy, 209, 210, 212, 213
Oesophagus, 175, 209–213
Oestrogens, 169
Ointments
  Canesten, 23
  Dactacort, 23
  Locoid, 23
  Terracortril, 24
  Triadcortyl, 23
Olfactory epithelium, 141
Operations
  Dohlman, 211
  Heller's, 210
  Schwartze, 38, 57
Opticrom (SCG), 156
Oracle, 119
Organ of corti, 66, 69, 106, 141
Organisations (for the deaf), 120
Organisms, anaerobic, 186
Oro-antral fistula, 149
Oropharynx, 175, 183
Osler's disease, see Hereditary telangiectasia
Ossicles (auditory),
  incus, 26, 27, 68
  malleus, 26, 27, 68
  stapes, 26, 27, 88
Ossicular chain and hearing, 69
Osteitis, 149
Osteomyelitis, 149
Otalgia (earache), 32
Otic capsule, 87
Otitic barotrauma, 59, 60
Otitis
  externa, 16, 17, 22, 23, 53, 58, 116
  postauricular, 17
Otitis media, 134, 142, 148, 196
  chemical, 29
Otitis media, acute
  bacteriology, 30
  clinical picture, 32
  complications, 36
  diagnosis, 32
  epidemiology, 29
  incidence, 28
  management, 32, 33, 34, 35, 46

natural history, 31
pathogenesis, 29
virology, 30
see also 85, 141
Otitis media, chronic suppurative, 37, 50–58, 102
  attico-antral, 50
  psychological aspects of, 58
  tubo-tympanic, 50
Otitis media, non-suppurative, see Glue ear and Otitis media, serous
Otitis media, recurrent, 36, 37
Otitis media, secretory, see Glue ear and Otitis media, serous
Otitis media, serous, 136
  see also Glue ear
Otolith membrane (organ), 65, 128
Otorrhoea (discharge), 22, 49, 50, 58
Otosclerosis, 87–91, 92, 123, 127
Otoscope, electric, 5, 6, 7, 9, 90
Otoscopy, 32
Otospongiosis, 87
Otosporin, 49
Ototoxic drugs, 33, 86, 103, 122, 127
Oval window, 27, 63, 94, 105
  rupture, 102
Oxygen
  absorption in middle ear, 31, 41
  concentration and ciliary action, 136
  in acute laryngo-tracheo-bronchitis, 202
Oxymetazoline (Iliadin-mini, Afrazine), 154
Oxytetracycline, 35

Paget's disease, 92
Palate, 133
  cleft, 41
  soft, 153, 175
Palsy
  bulbar, 208
  facial, 52
  vocal cord, 204, 205
Pansinusitis, 143
Papillary hypertrophic sinusitis, 147
Papillomata, laryngeal, 204
Paracetamol, 142
Paracusis, 88
Paradise, J. L., 37, 196
Paraffin, 166
Parasympathetic stimulation, 161
Paul Bunnell test, 188
Peak clipping, 115
Penicillins, 33, 34, 35, 102, 123, 142, 199, 200
  penicillin 'G', 37, 102, 192
  penicillin 'V', 35, 191

'Percentage disablement', 100, 101.
Perennial rhinitis, 157
Periapical abscess, 143
Perilymph, 63, 66, 90, 92, 102
Perilymph leak from round or oval window rupture, 102
Periodontitis, 143
Permanent threshold shift, 97
Petrositis, 38, 52
Petrous temporal bone, 38, 53, 63, 86, 145
pH, 136
Phagocytes, 152
Phagocytosis, 178
Pharyngitis, 141, 148
Pharynx, 175–179
  examination-children, 182
Phenylpropanolamine, 155
Phonation, 185
Pill (contraceptive), 91
Pinna
  anatomy, 15, 16
  congenital malformations, 18
  embryology, 18
  function, 68
Pistol shooting, 99
Placebo, 96
Plexus
  Auerbach's, 210
  tympanic, 27
Pneumonia, 140
Poliomyelitis, 140
Politzer, 87
Politzerisation, 45
Pollen, 152, 153, 154
Pollen counts, 153
Pollinex, 156
Polyarthritis, 141
Polycythemia, 86, 103, 193
Polymixins, 33
Polypi
  nasal, 139, 144, 145, 157, 158, 163–164
  of vocal cords, 204
Polypoid sinusitis, 147
Pop concerts, 99
Positional tests, 128–129
Post-aural aids, 112, 113
Posterior nares, 133
Posterior pharyngeal wall, 133
Post-nasal drip, 148
Post-nasal mirror, 12, 137
Pouch, pharyngeal, 210, 211
Powder
  boric acid and iodine, 23
  chloramphenicol, 23

Cicatrin, 23, 57
clotrimazole (Canesten), 23
Practice nurse, 74, 158
Prednisolone, 102
Prednisolone aqueous suspension (Deltastab), 155
Prednisone, 104
Pregnancy termination for maternal rubella, 81
Prematurity, 81
Presbycusis, 100, 104–107, 118
  management, 107
  pathology, 105–106
  types, 106
'Prescribed' occupations, 100
Prestel, 119
Private hearing aid dispenser, 112
Probe, Jobson Horne, 8, 9, 19
Prochlorperazine (Stemetil), 95, 127
Progesterone-only contraceptive, 91
Promontary, 27
Prostaglandins, 41
Pseudoephedrine, 155
Pseudomonas, 34
Pyocoele, 149
Pyramid, 26

Quinine, 86
Quinsy, 191, 196, 206

Radio aids, 85
Radioallergosorbent test (RAST), 158–159
Radiography (in nasal injuries), 170
Radiology, sinuses, 145
Radiotherapy, 206, 212, 213
  causing deafness, 102
  causing vocal cord palsy, 205
Ranitidine, (Zantac), 210
'Rat race', 161
Rebound vasodilatation, 154
Recessive inheritance of sensorineural deafness, 81
Recruitment, 70, 107, 109
Reflex, stapedius, 43, 45, 46–47
Rehabilitation of the deaf, 108, 110
Reissner's membrane, 66, 67, 93
Reserpine, 161
Reticulo-endothelial system, 178
Rhesus incompatibility, 81
Rheumatism, acute, 196
Rhinitis, 140, 148
  acute, 143
  allergic, 144, 152–160
  chronic, 146, 147–150
  chronic hypertrophic, 160

224 INDEX

Rhinitis (Cont'd)
  medicamentosa, 154
  non-allergic perennial, 160
  vasomotor, 152–162
Rhinorrhoea (nasal discharge), 141, 143, 148, 152, 153, 154, 157, 161–162
Rhinoscopy
  anterior, 136, 145, 148, 158, 164
  posterior, 136, 148, 164
Rifampin, 33, 34
Rifle shooting, 99
Rinne's test, 72, 88, 90
Road traffic accidents, 85
Round window, 27, 63, 66, 67, 69
  rupture, 102
Royal National Institute for the Deaf, 120
Rubella, 81
  immunisation at school, 82
  rubella antibody titre, 82
  rubella vaccine, 82
Rynacrom (SCG), 156

Saccule, 63, 64, 65, 66, 94, 124
  macula of, 66, 124, 125
Saccus drainage operations, 96
Saccus endolymphaticus, 63, 64, 96
Sadé, J., 45, 197
Salicylates, 45
Scala
  media (syn. cochlear duct), 63–66, 69, 92, 93
  tympani, 66, 69
  vestibuli, 66, 69
Scarlatina, 188
School teachers, 138
Seasonal rhinitis, 157
Semicircular canals, 63, 64, 65, 66, 124, 128
  ampulla, 65, 66, 128
  crista, 65, 66
  cupola, 65, 66
Semon's law, 205
Sensorineural hearing loss
  causes in children, 81
  in otosclerosis, 90
Sensory neuro-epithelium, 63
Septal deviations, 139
Septicaemia, 86
Serc (betahistine), 95
Serotonin, 153
Shea, J. J., 89
Sickle cell anaemia, 165
Sign, Schwartze's, 87

Silage, 153
Silver nitrate, 167, 169
Simpson's bag (tampon), 166, 167
Singers' nodes, 203–204
Single non-discriminating response of Douek, 141
Sinus agenesis, 145
Sinus baratrauma, 145
Sinuses (and ethmoid air cells), 134, 138
  ethmoid, 134, 163
  frontal, 133
  maxillary, 143, 163
  sphenoid, 133, 134
Sinusitis, 134, 141, 142, 157
  acute, 143–147
  chronic 147–150
Skin rashes, 141
Skin testing, 154, 158–159
Skull, base, 175
Sleep apnoea, 171, 193, 194
Small arms fire, 99
Smoking, 144, 182, 203
  see also, Tobacco, 212, 213
Sneezing, 152, 154, 157, 161
  and perilymph leak, 102
Snoring, 171, 195
Social worker, 111
Sodium cromoglycate (SCG), 155, 156
Sodium fluoride, 90
Sound level meter, 98
Soundproofing, 98, 110
Sound-proof room, 73, 121
Space
  post nasal, 26, 137, 163, 167
  subarrhachnoid, 66
Speaking tube, 107, 117
Specific neutralising antibodies, 139
Spectacle aids, 113
Speculum, Seigle's, 10, 42, 54
Speech discrimination, 106, 118
Speech frequencies, 100, 107, 111
Speech therapist, therapy, 204, 205
Spheno-ethmoid recess, 134
Spiral ganglion, 68, 106, 107
Spirochaeta denticulata, 188
Spray
  cocaine, 136, 158, 164, 166, 169, 183
  xylocaine, 164, 169, 183, 192
Stapedectomy, 88, 89, 90, 91
  complication, 90
  counselling, 91
Stapedial otosclerosis, 88
Stapes, 26, 27, 88
Stapes footplate, 63, 88
Stapes mobilisation operation, 89

Staphylococcus
  aureus, 34, 186
  pyogenes, 23, 31, 34
Statoconia, 65, 66
Stemetil, 95
Stereocilia, 124
Steroids (corticosteroids), 36, 45, 103, 104, 123, 155, 164, 202, 209
  dexamethasone, 201
Streptococcal infection, 196
Streptococcus
  anaerobic, 34
  Griffith's type, 4, 12, 25, 189
  group 'A', 186, 188, 191
  group 'B', 186
  group 'C', 186
  group 'G', 186
  haemolyticus, 186
  non-pathogenic, 191
  pneumoniae, 31, 34, 35, 37, 144
  type M5, 189
Streptomycin, 103
Stria vascularis, 66, 67, 106
Stricture, oesophageal, 208, 210, 211
Stridor, 199, 210, 202, 203
  in infants, 202
Striola, 124
Stugeron (Cinnarizine), 95
Sub-mucosa (of nose), 134
Submucosal diathermy, 162
Sudden sensorineural hearing loss, 101–104, 141
Sudden vestibular failure, see Failure, sudden vestibular
Sulcus, tympanic, 26
Sulphonamides, 33
Summating potential, 78
Superior olive, 77
Supraglottitis, 201
Surgery
  carotid endarterectomy, 205
  laser, 206
  thyroid, 205
Sweat test, 163
Swimming
  and grommets, 49
  and sinusitis, 144
Sympathetic stimulation, 160–161
Symphony orchestra players, 99
Syphilis, 81, 86, 92, 102, 123
Syphilisserological tests, 102
Syringe
  Bacon, 20
  Shaw's 20, 73
  Wood, 20

Tartrazines, 159
Tectorial membrane, 66, 67
Tegmen tympani, 27, 38
Telangectasia, hereditary, see Hereditary telangectasia
Teletext, 119
Television, 109, 118
Temporary threshold shift, 97
Teratogenic drugs, 81
Terfenadine (Triludan), 154
Tetracosactrin (Synacthen), 155
Tetracycline, 33, 34, 86, 142
Throat swabs, 188, 200
  significance, 186, 190, 191, 195, 196
Thrombocytopoenic purpura, 165
Thrombosis
  cavernous sinus, 149
  coronary, 167
  lateral sinus, 38, 52, 53
  posterior inferior cerebellar, 94, 95, 208
Thudichum's speculum, 9, 10, 136, 166
Ticarcillin, 33
Timothy grass, 153
Tinnitus, 59, 60, 68, 88, 91, 94, 99, 103, 107, 120–124
Tinnitus masker, 123, 124
Tobramycin., 34, 103
Tolerance of noise, 97
Tongue, base of, 175
Tongue depressors, 11, 12
Tonsil (faucial), 140, 175, 176, 177
Tonsil (lingual), 175, 177, 178
Tonsillectomy, 193, 195–196, 197
  mortality from, 195
Tonsillitis, 141, 148
  acute, 186–192
    aetiology, 186
    age incidence, 187
    clinical appearance, 186
    complications, 191
    diagnosis, 188
    differential diagnosis, 188
    management, 189
  chronic, 191
Toxaemia of pregnancy, 81
Toxins, 178
Toxoplasmosis, 81
Trachea, 138, 184, 185
Tracheitis, 141
Tracheostomy, 201, 202, 205, 208
Transillumination, 145
Triamcinolone aqueous suspension (Kenalog), 155
Trichloracetic acid, 169

Trismus, 192
Tubes
  emergency laryngostomy, 207
  endotracheal, trauma from, 182
  nasogastric, 208, 209
  Owen's, 213
Tubulin, 134
TUC policy, 110
Tullio phenomenon,
Tumour cerebral, 126
Tuning fork, 36, 72, 90
Tuning fork tests, 42, 72, 88, 107
Turbinates, 133, 134, 137, 139, 160–162
  inferior, 133, 148, 158
  middle, 133, 134, 169
  superior, 133, 163
Tympanic membrane
  anatomy, 26
  compliance, 43
  and hearing, 69
  infection, 25
  perforation, 21, 29, 31, 36, 50, 54
  retraction pocket, 52, 54
  secondary, 27, 66
  traumatic perforation, 59
Tympanogram, 43, 46–47
  see also, 39, 40
Tympanometry, 43, 44
  see also, 39
Tympanoplasty, 54
  combined approach, 56
Type I immediate hypersensitivity reaction, 152, 155
Type III delayed hypersensitivity reaction, 152, 155
Tyrosine absorbed vaccine, 156

Ulcers, contact (of vocal cords), 204
Underwater divers, 102
Unice, Dr. C., 124
Unidirectional microvalve, 96
Upper respiratory tract infections, 138–150, 165, 199, 201, 203
Utricle, 63, 65, 66, 124, 128
  macula, 65, 66, 124, 125
Uvulopalatopharyngoplasty, 171

Vaccine
  anti-D, 81
  pneumococcal, 31
Vacuum headache, 148
Vancomycin, 34
Vascular 'sludging', 103
Vasoconstrictor drops, 158, 166

Vasodilator drugs, 95, 103
Ventilated inserts (hearing aid), 116
Ventilating tubes, 45
Verbal communication, 80
Vernon, J., 123
Vertigo, 60, 88, 91, 103, 122, 124–129
Vertebrobasillar insufficiency, 126
Vestibular nuclei, 126
Vestibular neuronitis, see Sudden vestibular failure
Vestibule, inner ear, 63, 64
Vidian neurectomy, 162
Viraemia, 140
Viral infection (disease), 128, 138, 186, 205
Viruses, 127, 141
  corona, 138, 139
  Coxsackie, 139, 140, 144, 186
  echo, 139, 140, 144
  enteroviruses, 139
  influenza, 30, 40, 127, 140
  para-influenzal, 139, 140, 144, 186, 201
  respiratory syncitial, 30, 40, 139, 144, 201
  rhinoviruses, 138, 139, 144, 186
Vitamin C, 142
Vocabulary, 80
Volume control (hearing aid), 116, 118
Vomiting, 91, 94, 127

Waldeyer's ring, 175, 177, 178, 197
Wave, travelling, 69
Wax, 19, 85, 107
  hearing loss from, 71
  hook, 8, 9, 24
  removal, 19, 20, 21, 118
  solvents, 21, 85
  syringing, 20, 36
Web, oesophageal, 211, 212
Weber's test, 73
Whisper tests, 36, 42, 72, 90
White sound, 75
Wick, gauze, 24
Wilde's incision, 38
Wisbey, Dr. A., 42
Wood, Prof. C. B. S.,
  criteria for tonsillectomy, 195
Woodwind players, 99

X-Rays
  barium, 208, 209, 210, 211, 212, 213
  tomography, 94
Xylometazoline (Otrivine), 154